*Dementia with Lewy Bodies and
Parkinson's Disease Dementia*

Other Books by Dr. Ahlskog

The Parkinson's Disease Treatment Book

Partnering with your Doctor to Get the Most from Your Medications

Parkinson's Disease Treatment Guide for Physicians

Dementia with Lewy Bodies and Parkinson's Disease Dementia

Patient, Family, and Clinician Working
Together for Better Outcomes

J. ERIC AHLSKOG, PhD, MD

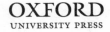

OXFORD
UNIVERSITY PRESS

Oxford University Press is a department of the University of Oxford.
It furthers the University's objective of excellence in research,
scholarship, and education by publishing worldwide.

Oxford New York
Auckland   Cape Town   Dar es Salaam   Hong Kong   Karachi
Kuala Lumpur   Madrid   Melbourne   Mexico City   Nairobi
New Delhi   Shanghai   Taipei   Toronto

With offices in
Argentina   Austria   Brazil   Chile   Czech Republic   France   Greece
Guatemala   Hungary   Italy   Japan   Poland   Portugal   Singapore
South Korea   Switzerland   Thailand   Turkey   Ukraine   Vietnam

Oxford is a registered trademark of Oxford University Press in the
UK and certain other countries.

Published in the United States of America by
Oxford University Press
198 Madison Avenue, New York, NY 10016

© Oxford University Press 2014

Library of Congress Cataloging-in-Publication Data
Ahlskog, J. Eric.
Dementia with Lewy bodies and Parkinson's disease dementia : patient, family, and clinician
working together for better outcomes / J. Eric Ahlskog, Ph.D., M.D.
pages cm
Includes bibliographical references and index.
ISBN 978-0-19-997756-7
1. Parkinson's disease—Chemotherapy.   2. Lewy body dementia—Chemotherapy.
3. Patient compliance.   I. Title.
RC382.A364 2013
616.8'33—dc23
2013006243

Table of Contents

Preface   ix

Acknowledgments   xv

INTRODUCTION TO DEMENTIA WITH LEWY
BODIES AND PARKINSON'S DISEASE DEMENTIA

1   Background   3

2   What Is Known about the Cause   15

3   Are There Medications for Slowing Disease Progression?   19

4   Symptoms, Related Brain Regions, and Diagnosis   25

TREATMENT

LEVODOPA-RESPONSIVE PROBLEMS

5   Which Drug for Parkinsonism? Walking, Stiffness,
Tremor, and Slowness   49

6   Beginning Carbidopa/Levodopa Treatment:
Background, Starting Dosages, and Side Effects   61

7   Parkinsonism Treatment for Those
Already on Medications   81

8   Unstable Responses and Dyskinesias: Later
Motor Problems   89

9 Other Levodopa-Responsive Problems: Anxiety,
   Insomnia, and Pain   101

PROBLEMS CAUSED OR EXACERBATED BY
PARKINSON MEDICATIONS

10 Hallucinations and Delusions   111

11 Pathologic Behaviors Provoked by Dopamine
    Agonist Drugs: Gambling, Sex, Eating, and Spending   117

COGNITIVE PROBLEMS

12 Dementia: Impaired Thinking and
    Judgment; Confusion   125

DYSAUTONOMIA: BLOOD PRESSURE,
BLADDER, BOWELS

13 Blood Pressure and Orthostatic Hypotension:
    Faints, Near-Faints, and Lightheadedness   141

14 Bladder Problems   161

15 Bowels and Constipation   169

OTHER SLEEP PROBLEMS

16 Daytime Drowsiness   177

17 Acting Out Dreams: REM Sleep Behavior Disorder   193

MORE GENERAL ISSUES

18 Depression   199

19 General Medical Issues   207

20 Benefits of Regular Exercise: Disease-Slowing?   217

21 Hospitalization and Nursing Facilities:
    Keeping Everyone on the Same Page   231

22 Families, Caregivers, and Assistance   237

    Glossary   245

    Index   251

Preface

This book focuses on two Lewy body disorders, dementia with Lewy bodies and Parkinson's disease with dementia. The target audience includes patients, spouses, partners, family members, and especially caregivers. Although written for a lay audience, clinicians and the entire health care team should also find this book very helpful.

The spectrum of dementia is broad in these Lewy body conditions. In some individuals dementia may be mild and relatively stable; for these people this book may be a very useful read. For others with these illnesses it is the caregivers who need help understanding the myriad problems and how to treat them. This book targets a broad audience. Most readers will not be familiar with medical words or concepts. It is hoped that this book will communicate the many important messages in easily understood terms.

Affected people leaving the doctor's office with a diagnosis of dementia with Lewy bodies or Parkinson's disease with dementia are often confused by these terms and their implications. These are not familiar diagnoses, nor are *Lewy bodies* part of our everyday language. Even the term *dementia* is easily misinterpreted. For some, this implies a zombie-like state at the end of life. However, the term has broad meanings and does not necessarily imply the end of useful life, or of hope.

Why are these two disorders combined in this book? And what in the world are Lewy bodies? The answers to those questions should become apparent in Chapter 1, but let me briefly provide an overview.

Lewy bodies are microscopic accumulations of specific proteins within brain cells, which are the hallmark of Parkinson's disease. With advanced Parkinson's disease, this Lewy process presumably spreads to involve the highest brain regions that are the centers for thinking and memory. The condition is then called Parkinson's disease with dementia. Restated, what was initially simple Parkinson's disease later became complicated with dementia. In contrast, dementia with Lewy bodies is associated with early widespread distribution of this Lewy process throughout the brain. In this disorder, the thinking and memory problems are present at the outset. Under the microscope, these two conditions look the same. Thus, scientists debate whether dementia with Lewy bodies is essentially the same condition as advanced Parkinson's disease with dementia.

These two disorders are often treated by specialists from two different disciplines: dementia specialists often diagnose and treat those with dementia with Lewy bodies; conversely, movement disorder specialists often care for those who have Parkinson's disease with dementia. This may lead to diverging ideas about how best to treat the disorder. In this book, the object is to synthesize therapeutic advice and keep it as simple as possible.

The primary goal of this book is optimal treatment. Arming patients and families with crucial facts and principles will better enable them to work in tandem with the treating doctors. As a team, they can then work together to optimize medications and avoid troublesome drug interactions.

These Lewy conditions are associated with a myriad of component problems, ranging from hallucinations or insomnia to walking difficulties. Although there is no cure, many of these problems lend themselves to treatment. Moreover, some problems are made worse by inadvertent administration of drugs for other symptoms. These treatment options sometimes become complex, even for savvy clinicians. Knowledgeable patients and family members can be an invaluable ally to the clinician.

For many people with these Lewy conditions an important component of their disability is impaired standing, walking, and movement. This is the "parkinsonism" component, and it often responds quite dramatically to treatment. However, some of the medications used may cause more problems than benefits. Hence, portions of this book address common medication side effects in detail. It is easy to veer off on the wrong track without this knowledge. Again, a teamwork approach is desired.

Why bother to do this? In the old days, patients received immutable instructions from their doctor in terse terms: "take one pill three times a day," end of story. Back then, medical science was not very advanced, and the medicines were limited. Since then, medical knowledge has grown exponentially and with it a variety of medications. In fact, there are so many drugs that they often interact with one another. Just keeping the drug names straight can be a challenge. In this book the brand names of drugs are capitalized and listed between parentheses after the generic form.

Complicating medical care are the modest fixed reimbursements for office visits in the United States. The government and insurance agencies have concluded that face-to-face counseling about medical conditions and medications is not a highly valued service. Hence, primary care doctors, internists, and neurologists have negative incentives for spending time just talking with their patients. The doctor can explain and counsel as long as he or she would like; however, there is no reimbursement for this beyond a limited fee. This is why doctor visits tend to be brief and focused. However, those with these Lewy conditions have many complex problems that need to be addressed What is the solution to this conundrum? Certainly, arriving for the doctor appointment knowing the issues and treatment options is an important start. This can help streamline the discussion and help the doctor provide the best care.

In this book, we will cover all the major problems that occur in these Lewy disorders. While not everyone with these conditions experiences all of these problems, the intent here is to be comprehensive and address all possibilities. Since some of these problems may never develop, it is not important to closely scrutinize every chapter. However, it would be wise to at least skim these so that if a problem eventually surfaces you will know where to find answers.

There is a broad spectrum of Lewy body severity, ranging from milder and treatable conditions to those individuals needing intensive caregiving and even nursing facilities. Advanced problems, caregiving, and collaboration with nurses in hospitals and homes is the focus near the end of this book.

What is the source of these treatment guidelines? The voluminous medical literature contains countless treatises about treatment, but conflicting opinions abound. Commercial revenue streams drive some of these discussions. In this book, the controversies have been adjudicated first and foremost by patients and family coming to the clinic. They are the ones who report responses to treatment. As a full-time Mayo Clinic neurologist for over 30 years, I have had the privilege of caring for many such patients, and they have taught me much. This experience has proven to be a valuable resource and the basis for many of the guidelines provided in this book.

I often am asked to speak at patient and family Lewy conferences, and I especially welcome questions from the audience. The general approach that I take in this book is similar to my responses to questions after lectures. I cannot become someone's doctor from a distance, but I can relate how I would address someone's problem if they were in my clinic. My intention is to open up avenues of thought and discussion. Possible alternative strategies to treating a current problem can be raised with the primary physician as appropriate. The primary clinician must be the captain of the team, but broad thinking can only be good. Please use this book as a starting point in discussion with your clinical team.

JEA

Acknowledgments

I wish to single out two mentors who were crucial to my academic and medical career: Professor Mark Rilling, Michigan State University, and Professor Bartley Hoebel, Princeton University. They were role models, and they opened crucial avenues for subsequent steps in my academic life. I am also grateful for the good fortune to have found my way to the Mayo Clinic, where the phrase "patients come first" guides practice. My 30 years on staff at Mayo in Rochester, Minnesota has been a truly extraordinary experience, and I treasure my Mayo colleagues who have taught me much. Growing up in the Midwest, I anticipated adult life in a warmer climate, later discovering that the quality of life in Minnesota easily offsets the winters.

I also wish to take this opportunity to assuage long-standing, personal guilt for an extremely belated statement of gratitude. This goes to my high school teachers who overcame remarkable challenges, defying odds to prepare me (and my classmates) for the academic and real-life opportunities that lay ahead. Unfortunately, these teachers have now all passed on. Their importance in my life will become apparent as I put this into context.

The last half of my youth was spent in small-town America: Kaleva, Michigan, population 385. My grandparents had located their farm there a century ago and raised nine children.

I was born in Chicago and moved to Kaleva after my father died when I was finishing grade school. Like many rural, small-town schools, Kaleva High School (KHS) was barely supported by tax revenues and had been threatened with condemnation for failing to maintain building codes. Despite upgrades that met code, it was later to be torn down shortly after my high school graduation. The challenges to the KHS teaching staff were enormous. Prototypic was Mr. Ebert, who taught all the science and math classes to every Kaleva high school grade level all day, every day. I had him for freshman biology and algebra; sophomore chemistry and geometry; junior physics; and senior advanced mathematics. In retrospect, this daily teaching load seems incredible, if not impossible, so I will reiterate. Each day, all high school freshmen through seniors had the following classes taught by him: algebra, biology, chemistry (plus lab), physics (plus lab), geometry and advanced math. Also exemplary was my high school basketball, baseball, and track coach, Mr. Sturm. Besides coaching all sports (junior varsity and varsity), he also taught me freshman typing, sophomore marketing, and junior accounting and was the high school principal. He also taught me eighth-grade science my first year in Kaleva.

One teacher, Mr. Main, taught all the history, geography, economics, and social science courses to all grades. Fortunately for us, Mr. Main presciently recognized the historical era in which we were living, which included the Nixon-Kennedy debates, the Cuban missile crisis and Kennedy Camelot. In lieu of books, we read *Time* magazine and debated current affairs. Despite living in such a rural community, we became citizens of the world and ongoing students of history, as we continued to live through a remarkable era.

This book is written with complete sentences, including subjects, verbs, and appropriate punctuation. This skill is owed to Mr. Clift (English teacher), who would never be accused of undervaluing the role of diagramming sentences on the blackboard.

How did all these gifted and enthusiastic teachers come to a farming town of 385 people? Much of the credit must go to the superintendent, Mr. Hoeh, who found talent in unlikely places. When the school lost its English and social science teachers before my senior year, Mr. Hoeh recruited the town doctor's very smart but underutilized wife to teach social studies (Mrs. Seutter) and a retired, overqualified Presbyterian minister from a nearby town to teach English, Mr. Gehring.

What was the outcome? Obviously, I was able to graduate from college and beyond, plus medical school. However, more remarkable for our small town is that fact that all six boys in my high school class earned 4-year college degrees and became successful and accomplished citizens. Like the children of Lake Wobegon, we were apparently all above average.

Fast-forward now to my current role, helping to care for those with Parkinson's disease and Lewy body dementia. Patients have taught me nearly as much as text books. We have been partners, and I have benefitted enormously from what I have learned from my patients and their caregivers. I must acknowledge and thank them for their lessons conveyed to me. I have had the benefit of peering into the lives of countless families. I have been humbled by the thankless dedication to loved ones that is provided by spouses, partners, children, and other caregivers. Couples in my clinic have shown me the true meaning of love. As we converse in my clinic, I often try to imagine the couple as they were decades before. What did they look like when first courting and enjoying their youth? Now, as they have grown older together, the declining health of one burdens the other. Yet, I have realized that for many, the burden is assumed with continuing love and commitment; sometimes the love is unrequited due to the problems of dementia. How discouraging it must be for the spouse when that handsome young man, once ready to conquer the world, is no longer able to walk or converse well, or when the lovely woman who raised a family and attended to everyone else's needs can no longer care for herself. The love I have seen in the clinic provided by spouses, partners, and children continues to inspire me, and daily renews my faith in our humanity.

I thank Joan Bossert, Vice President/Editorial Director of Brain and Behavioral Sciences at Oxford University Press, who has supported and encouraged me as I wrote my first book for people with Parkinson's disease and now this book for people with Lewy conditions affecting memory and thinking. Joan edited my first book, tactfully conveying the importance of a succinct and nonredundant text. Those lessons were invaluable in writing the current book.

Where did I find the time for writing? My lovely and long-suffering wife, Faye, has not complained (recently) when I repeatedly came home late and was gone weekend mornings. She continues to lovingly support me, and without that, none of this would have been possible. To Faye and my wonderful three sons, Mike, John, and Matt: I feel truly blessed for your support and love.

INTRODUCTION TO DEMENTIA WITH LEWY BODIES AND PARKINSON'S DISEASE DEMENTIA

1

Background

This book has a combined focus on two neurodegenerative conditions: dementia with Lewy bodies and Parkinson's disease with dementia. While patients with either disorder experience quite variable problems, these two disorders have striking similarities when viewed in the aggregate. Thus, the symptoms of these two conditions are much the same, and so are the treatment strategies.

Before addressing treatment, it is crucial to define the relevant terms, broaden our understanding, and discuss how these diagnoses are made. We will start with some basics.

WHAT ARE NEURODEGENERATIVE CONDITIONS?

These disorders typically start in middle age and later, where selected brain circuits deteriorate for unknown reasons. Common neurodegenerative conditions include Parkinson's disease, Alzheimer's disease, and amyotrophic lateral sclerosis (ALS; Lou Gehrig's disease). Such conditions involve limited regions of the brain or spinal cord, slowly progressing and leading to disability. Each is clinically identified by the specific neurologic deficits unique to that condition. Why each affects certain brain regions, sparing others, is a crucial but unanswered question. Although much has been learned about degenerative syndromes, we do not know the causes of any of them.

WHAT IS DEMENTIA?

Dementia implies a loss of intellectual abilities sufficient to compromise activities of daily living. Most often the term *dementia* is used in the context of neurodegenerative disorders. Mild thinking and memory problems that do not substantially interfere with daily routines fall into the category of mild cognitive impairment (MCI; see below).

Doctors diagnosing dementia rely on the history from the patient and family, plus cognitive tests. Short tests assessing memory, attention, and calculation, among other things, can be done in the doctor's office. Such tests include the so-called Mini-Mental State Examination and the Short Test of Mental Status. More refined and informative tests, termed psychometric testing, are done under the auspices of psychologists; these typically require 2 to 4 hours.

Clinicians addressing dementia must also look for treatable causes before concluding that the problem is a neurodegenerative dementia. This assessment typically includes a brain scan, blood tests, and a review of the patient's medical history and medication list, which may indicate the need for additional testing.

While Alzheimer's disease is the most common cause of neurodegenerative dementia, there are a variety of other neurodegenerative conditions that can cause dementia, including dementia with Lewy bodies (DLB) and Parkinson's disease with dementia (PDD). DLB and PDD do not affect cognition in the same way as Alzheimer's disease (discussed later in this chapter).

MILD COGNITIVE IMPAIRMENT (MCI)

Modest intellectual impairment that does not impair activities of daily living is not dementia; however, it might be a forerunner of dementia. That is called "mild cognitive impairment," a term coined by the Mayo dementia specialist, Dr. Ronald Petersen. *Cognition* refers to thinking, memory, perception, judgment, and intellectual function in general. The distinction of those with MCI from those with dementia should be especially important in the future when we have drugs to treat the cause or causes of MCI; early treatment would then be crucial.

WHAT ARE LEWY BODIES?

Lewy bodies are the hallmarks of both DLB and PDD when brain tissue is examined under the microscope. Lewy bodies were recognized years ago as microscopic markers of Parkinson's disease, as depicted in Figure 1.1.

The Lewy body story goes back nearly a century, when Dr. Fredric Lewy described small clumps of matter within brain cells (neurons) among people who died with Parkinson's disease. Subsequently, these neuron inclusions were found to be universal in the lower end of the brain (brain stem) in people with Parkinson's disease. To this day, microscopic

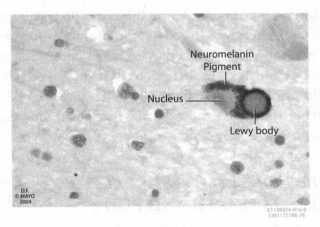

Figure 1.1 Microscopic picture of a Lewy body within a neuron (brain cell). This neuron is within the substantia nigra and contains neuromelanin pigment, which is normal for this cell.

Lewy bodies are accepted as confirmation of a diagnosis of Parkinson's disease, although visualizing brain Lewy bodies is not possible in life.

Only in the last 20 to 25 years have Lewy bodies been acknowledged as marking certain other dementing disorders. Researchers came to recognize that not all dementia is Alzheimer's disease, with the second leading cause of dementia being DLB. In this disorder, Lewy bodies were found microscopically in brain regions responsible for cognition. Subsequently, it was recognized that people who initially had simple Parkinson's disease but later developed dementia also displayed widespread microscopic Lewy bodies in cognitive brain regions.

To summarize, Lewy bodies are now regarded as the hallmark of not only Parkinson's disease but also DLB and PDD. The way in which these conditions relate to one another, and whether there are common causes, is open to speculation.

Lewy bodies cannot be seen under the microscope unless the brain tissue is properly prepared and special stains are used. The most sensitive indicator of Lewy bodies involves an antibody stain that specifically binds to a naturally occurring brain protein called alpha synuclein. This alpha synuclein stain selectively labels Lewy bodies. Using these sensitive staining techniques, researchers recognized that clumps of this substance are found not only in the cell bodies of these brain cells (neurons) but also in the extensions of brain cells (axons); such clumping might impair neuron function and brain signaling. We will discuss alpha synuclein in more detail in Chapter 2, since this may have important implications for the cause of these conditions.

OTHER CONTRIBUTIONS TO THE DEMENTIA OF DLB AND PDD

The dementia of both DLB and PDD is due to the Lewy body neurodegenerative process. However, three other factors also contribute, to varying degrees. By themselves, these other three factors are not the primary causes of dementia in Lewy conditions but are additive; they each reduce the threshold for dementia if Lewy neurodegeneration is ongoing. One such factor is cerebrovascular disease, which may manifest as stroke (large or small). Cerebrovascular disease may be unrecognized; it may also manifest as brain atherosclerosis (hardening of the arteries). Atherosclerosis of small brain arteries is the reason for leukoaraiosis, which is the white blush present to varying extents on the magnetic resonance imaging (MRI) brain scans of older adults. Treating risk factors for such cerebrovascular disease, especially earlier in life, is wise; however, once dementia is present it may be too late. Such risk factors include hypertension, diabetes mellitus, elevated cholesterol, smoking, and lack of exercise.

A second contributor to dementia, but not a major factor in DLB or PDD, is Alzheimer brain pathology—i.e., the same brain microscopic changes seen in people with Alzheimer's disease. Such microscopic changes slowly accumulate with aging in most humans, even those without dementia. In many older adults they are modest and not sufficient to result in dementia. However, in a brain already challenged with Lewy neurodegenerative pathology, there is little reserve; a small degree of brain Alzheimer pathology will be additive. Such changes are noted in many, but not all, with DLB or PDD.

Finally, contributing to the dementia of DLB and PDD is normal brain aging. With passing decades of life our brains shrink, which is very apparent on MRI brain scans in those over age 80 years. This is primarily due to loss of brain connections as part of the aging process. Although there is a modest, age-related loss of brain cells (neurons), the primary reason for brain shrinkage is loss of synapses and the connecting neuron circuitry (axon terminals, portions of dendrites). Fortunately, many older adults without Alzheimer's or Lewy disease are able to compensate for this age-related brain shrinkage, but it is additive if neurodegenerative disorders are present.

WHAT IS PARKINSON'S DISEASE AND HOW IS THIS RELEVANT TO DEMENTIA WITH LEWY BODIES?

As we have learned, the Lewy body is the microscopic brain-marker of Parkinson's disease. Some people with Parkinson's disease later develop dementia, and it appears that this reflects the spread of the Lewy neurodegenerative process to cognitive regions of the brain. When this occurs, it is termed Parkinson's disease with dementia (PDD). Not everyone with Parkinson's disease will become demented; however, the risk becomes substantial among those with very long disease durations and survival to an older age.

The German neuroanatomist Dr. Heikko Braak is credited with recognizing the spread of the Lewy process, which parallels the progression of Parkinson's disease. This occurs over many years. Thus, in early Parkinson's disease, the Lewy changes are largely confined to the lower brain stem, as depicted in Figure 1.2. However, Lewy neurodegeneration spreads from the lower brain stem slowly over many years to higher levels, ultimately to the cortex (see Figure 1.2); thought, perception,

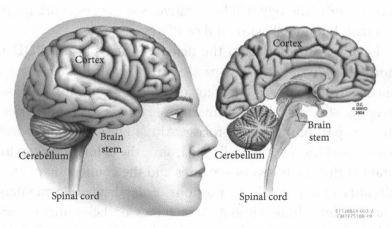

Figure 1.2 Illustration of human brain showing the brain stem and cortex.

and memory are primarily centered in the cortex. Involvement of the cortex is the primary basis for the dementia that develops later in some people with Parkinson's disease.

To recap: in Parkinson's disease, the Lewy neurodegenerative changes are restricted to limited brain regions (e.g., brain stem) while sparing higher centers necessary for thinking and memory (cortex). In PDD, the Lewy process has spread to cognitive brain areas. How and why this spread occurs is the subject of intensive scientific investigation.

Perhaps we should not be surprised that DLB has an almost identical microscopic appearance to that of PDD. By the time Parkinson's disease evolves to PDD, the symptoms are typically much the same as those of DLB. Under the microscope, even the most expert neuropathologists cannot distinguish the brain of those with DLB from a brain with PDD; in each, Lewy bodies abound in brain regions that are the substrate for thinking and memory. Restated, Parkinson's disease often evolves to PDD, and PDD is very similar to DLB, both symptomatically and under the microscope.

More on Parkinson's Disease

Since Parkinson's disease is so intimately connected to DLB and PDD, we need to consider this in more detail. There is a lot more to this brain story than the mere presence of Lewy bodies.

Classic symptoms of Parkinson's disease involve movement, including tremor, walking problems, stiffness (rigidity), and slowness (bradykinesia). Nearly 50 years ago it was discovered that these motor problems were associated with loss of a specific brain neurotransmitter, dopamine. A *neurotransmitter* is a signaling chemical that is released by individual neurons (brain cells), tending to activate or inhibit the next link in that brain circuit. Scientists reasoned that if brain dopamine is low, replenishment of brain dopamine should reverse symptoms. It was recognized that dopamine pills would not work, since dopamine has a chemical structure that will not allow it to enter the brain (i.e., it could not cross the natural barrier between the bloodstream and the brain, termed the blood–brain barrier). However, the natural precursor to dopamine, levodopa (L-dopa) is able to cross; levodopa is easily converted to dopamine by a native enzyme. This led to the development of an effective symptomatic treatment for Parkinson's disease, levodopa. This remains the most efficacious symptomatic medication for Parkinson's disease and is the foundation of treatment.

Dopamine deficiencies are also present in DLB, as well as in PDD. Subsequent chapters on treatment (Chapters 5–9) will address when and how dopamine replenishment is appropriate in those conditions.

What are the Symptoms of Parkinson's Disease?

Given the relationship between Parkinson's disease, PDD, and DLB, the specific condition of Parkinson's disease deserves further discussion. To varying degrees, the symptoms of Parkinson's disease are also present in DLB, as they are in PDD.

Movement problems are the primary symptoms of Parkinson's disease during the early years and sometimes for many years. As stated earlier, the classic motor symptoms include slowness of movement (bradykinesia), stiffness (rigidity), and often, but not always, a tremor. This tremor is unique in that it is present when the affected limb is relaxed; hence it is termed a "resting tremor." Finally, walking problems are typical of Parkinson's disease, especially a shuffling gait with reduced swinging of the arms. These symptoms are quite responsive to replenishment of brain dopamine with levodopa therapy (carbidopa/levodopa) or synthetic forms of dopamine, known as dopamine agonists (pramipexole, ropinirole, rotigotine, and apomorphine).

Non-motor symptoms are also a component of Parkinson's disease but often get less publicity. The autonomic nervous system is commonly affected by Lewy neurodegenerative processes. Autonomic symptoms may include constipation, urinary incontinence, or faintness due to low blood pressure when upright. Other symptoms commonly reported by people with Parkinson's disease include anxiety, depression, loss of smell, insomnia, and acting out dreams (REM sleep behavior disorder).

These Parkinson's disease symptoms are present to varying degrees in DLB. Occasionally, they are more problematic than the dementia.

Now that we have this background, we are in a position to better define and distinguish the disorders that are the focus of this book: DLB and PDD.

PARKINSON'S DISEASE WITH DEMENTIA (PDD)

Parkinson's disease is not a static condition, as we have just learned. One way that it progresses relates to the consistency of the levodopa response. Specifically, control of symptoms with levodopa therapy becomes less stable after a number of years. However, this is usually manageable, although not always perfectly. The more troublesome progression of the Lewy neurodegenerative process relates to the later development of cognitive impairment. The characteristics of this impairment are different from Alzheimer's disease, where memory is typically affected first and foremost. Sometimes, the cognitive symptoms of PDD are relatively mild and occasionally only very slowly progressive. However, they may also be quite prominent and troublesome. When that occurs, they mirror the problems of DLB, discussed next.

DEMENTIA WITH LEWY BODIES (DLB)

Dementia with Lewy bodies is the second leading cause of neurodegenerative dementia, second only to Alzheimer's disease.

DLB might be confused with Alzheimer's disease because they both affect cognition. They are, however, distinct conditions.

The cognitive problems of Alzheimer's disease are quite different from those of DLB. Memory is affected first and foremost in Alzheimer's disease, whereas other aspects of cognition are more likely to be impaired in DLB. Individuals with DLB typically have predominant difficulties with higher-level planning and organization (executive function), as well as visuospatial function (perception and conceptualization of two- and three-dimensional space). The cognitive profile of typical DLB will be discussed in more detail in Chapter 4. Moreover, DLB is usually associated with the movement problems of parkinsonism as well as some of the non-movement problems, such as loss of smell, autonomic dysfunction (constipation, urinary incontinence), or dream enactment behavior during sleep (REM sleep behavior disorder). The diagnosis of DLB becomes much more apparent when it takes on features of Parkinson's disease, but this may occur much later, delaying the diagnosis.

Under the microscope, the hallmark features of Alzheimer's disease are brain neuritic plaques and neurofibrillary tangles rather than Lewy bodies. The biochemical components of these plaques and tangles differ from those of Lewy bodies and suggest different causative mechanisms. It is true that some people with DLB also have limited numbers of these plaques and tangles, but they are overshadowed by Lewy bodies and related Lewy features. However, this occasional overlap has led scientists to question whether the development of one condition somehow triggers the other in some individuals.

In any case, DLB and Alzheimer's disease are fundamentally different disorders. Although the microscopic changes cannot be known in life, the character of the dementia and the associated features typically allow the clinician to make a correct diagnosis.

WHY AND HOW DO WE DISTINGUISH DLB FROM PDD?

This is a curious scenario of two conditions, DLB and PDD, which ultimately end up as largely the same disorder but by two different routes. PDD starts as Parkinson's disease, which then progresses to include dementia; those with DLB start out with dementia . Are these just different ends of a single spectrum? Are they really the same disorder? This is an unresolved question.

Once the fully developed clinical problems are present, how can these be distinguished? The answer lies in the clinical course. Parkinson's disease is devoid of intellectual problems when it first develops. In contrast, cognitive impairment is present at the onset of DLB, sometimes with parkinsonism delayed. In fact, some people with DLB never experience parkinsonism.

How do researchers make the distinction? When studying these conditions, strict definitions are necessary so that there is no confusion over what is being studied. An international consensus panel has instituted the so-called 1-year rule to separate DLB from PDD:

- If cognitive impairment is initially present or develops within the first clinical year of the Lewy disorder, this is termed *dementia with Lewy bodies*.
- If the initial clinical picture is Parkinson's disease without cognitive impairment and if intellectual decline develops after the first year, then this is termed *Parkinson's disease with dementia*.

This is a working rule and may be modified in the future as we gain greater understanding of these conditions. However, for practical therapeutic purposes, one can see why DLB and PDD would be addressed together in this book, focused on treatment.

2

What Is Known about the Cause

Most of the research into the cause of Lewy disorders has focused on Parkinson's disease, since that is the best defined of these conditions and, therefore, the most straightforward to study. Dementia with Lewy bodies (DLB) is more difficult to diagnose with certainty, especially in the early years of the disease. What we collectively learn about Parkinson's disease will likely be very relevant to our understanding of DLB.

Multiple investigations have linked Parkinson's disease to both environmental exposures and genetic factors. However, these associations have all been modest, and none of them accounts for more than a few percent of the contribution to the cause of sporadic Parkinson's disease (i.e., the attributable risks are low). These investigations are ongoing and hopefully will soon provide a more complete understanding of the cause(s).

Perhaps the most important clue to all Lewy conditions is located in the brain: the Lewy body itself. A recent sophisticated analysis of Lewy bodies revealed approximately 300 different component proteins. However, we already knew that Lewy bodies contain high concentrations of a normal protein called alpha synuclein. In fact, Lewy bodies are conventionally identified under the microscope with antibody stains that specifically bind to alpha synuclein. Could this be the crucial protein among the nearly 300?

THE ALPHA SYNUCLEIN STORY

While the alpha synuclein story is focused on Parkinson's disease, it may be just as relevant to DLB, as we shall see. The story starts with a large Italian-American family with Parkinson's disease, studied by Dr. Lawrence Golbe and colleagues at the Robert Wood Johnson Medical Center in New Brunswick, New Jersey. In this rare family, many members of multiple generations had been affected by Parkinson's disease (with Lewy bodies), consistent with a single gene passed on with dominant inheritance. It took a number of years to identify that abnormal gene, which ultimately was proven to be the gene coding for alpha synuclein. It was quickly discovered that this genetic error is not present in usual cases of Parkinson's disease. However, alpha synuclein is present in substantial amounts in Lewy bodies from all people with Parkinson's disease. A number of years later, an Iowa family with similar dominantly inherited Parkinson's disease was studied at the Mayo Clinic. Initial studies revealed that the alpha-synuclein gene code was normal. Dr. Matthew Farrer at Mayo Jacksonville ultimately recognized that the cause was not an error in the genetic code but an extra alpha-synuclein gene, producing excessive amounts of alpha synuclein. Dr. Farrer also discovered a similar mechanism in other families, including some in which dementia was early and prominent. Such early dementia was associated with carrying not just one, but two extra genes (triplication of the normal gene). In contrast, carrying only one extra gene (duplication) was associated with a less aggressive course, often without dementia (i.e., Parkinson's disease alone). Apparently, producing more alpha synuclein was detrimental.

Alpha-synuclein genetic coding has been extensively studied. These genetic abnormalities do not account for typical Parkinson's disease or routine DLB. However, minor variability in the normal genetic code for alpha synuclein appears to be a risk factor for Parkinson's disease. Specifically, normal differences in genetic coding (polymorphisms) that regulate how much alpha synuclein is produced influence the risk for developing Parkinson's disease, albeit modestly. Whether this is also true for DLB has not been studied.

HOW MIGHT ALPHA SYNUCLEIN BECOME PROBLEMATIC?

Alpha synuclein is a normal protein contained within brain cells (neurons). If it becomes toxic, why and how might this occur? The current explanation is that it appears to clump together (aggregate), apparently impairing normal degradation and disposal by brain cells. It is presumed that this aggregated alpha synuclein might interfere with the normal function of these neurons. Many investigators believe that the actual Lewy bodies may not be toxic per se but rather are a type of cellular garbage can where the neuron deposits cellular "junk." Presumably, the actual toxic products may be small aggregates that accumulate throughout the neuron and impede normal function. Thus, pathologists examining brains of those with Lewy disorders see not only Lewy bodies but also small strands (Lewy neurites) and tiny aggregate dots. It may be that these or even smaller collections are the problematic species. Investigators also speculate that the cellular disposal mechanisms for dealing with such protein collections may also play a role. If compromised, this might allow these aggregates to accumulate.

HOW DOES THE ALPHA-SYNUCLEIN HYPOTHESIS FIT WITH THE PROGRESSION OF LEWY DISORDERS?

The German neuroanatomist Professor Heikko Braak has proposed a plausible scheme to explain the progression of

Parkinson's disease evolving to dementia. Although dementia does not develop in everyone with Parkinson's disease, this is not a static condition, and over years, increasing problems of various types typically surface. The Braak scheme fits with the known characteristics of the Parkinson's disease brain when studied at various points in time. The earliest stage is associated with Lewy pathology limited to the lower brain stem and the organs of smell, the olfactory bulbs. At this early stage, Lewy bodies are also found outside the central nervous system in the autonomic nervous system (which regulates bowel and bladder function, and blood pressure). According to this scheme, the Lewy changes gradually advance forward in the brain. When the midbrain is reached, the dopamine-containing neurons in the substantia nigra are affected. Years later, the ascending progression may reach the cortex and related structures that are the substrates for cognition.

How and why does this progression occur? Professor Braak has hypothesized that there may be some product, perhaps alpha synuclein, that is slowly passed from neuron to neuron. With each new brain cell, seeding of the inciting substance could initiate the process.

Although this scheme is plausible for Parkinson's disease, including Parkinson's disease evolving to dementia, it does not adequately account for the clinical course of DLB. The symptoms of DLB suggest that Lewy pathology is already widespread within the brain when it is first clinically recognized. Moreover, some people with DLB do not have symptoms of brain stem (lower brain) involvement; for example, not everyone with DLB has parkinsonism. If the Braak scheme is to be applied to DLB, then one would need to hypothesize a more rapid but less destructive ascension through the brain. In other words, the Lewy process might progress more quickly throughout the brain but be relatively more destructive at higher (cognitive) levels. However, this is not an entirely satisfying explanation, and more research must be directed at these issues.

3

Are There Medications for Slowing Disease Progression?

If diagnosed with dementia with Lewy bodies (DLB) or Parkinson's disease, one would naturally want to do everything possible to halt or at least slow the disease progression. Are there medications for this purpose? Unfortunately, no controlled trials have analyzed this question among people with DLB. On the other hand, multiple randomized clinical trials have assessed a variety of drugs as possible agents to slow the progression of another Lewy disorder, Parkinson's disease. If a strategy were available to slow the progression of Parkinson's disease, that could be relevant to all Lewy conditions.

Major clinical trials assessing drugs to slow the progression of Parkinson's disease date back to the 1980s. In each of these trials hundreds of Parkinson's disease patients from multiple participating medical centers were enrolled and randomized to either the study drug or a placebo. Drugs that have been investigated included high doses of vitamin E; the monoamine oxidase B (MAO-B) inhibitor selegiline (deprenyl); the dopamine agonists pramipexole and ropinirole; as well as two experimental agents shown in animals to reduce apoptosis (a cell death process that might be relevant to neurodegeneration). Unfortunately, none of these large trials provided compelling evidence for slowing the progression of Parkinson's disease. The studies' results were either negative or so confounded and inconclusive that a meaningful interpretation could not be drawn.

Most recently, the newer MAO-B inhibitor rasagiline (which also reduces apoptosis) was similarly assessed in two large clinical trials. The outcomes from these rasagiline studies were mixed and difficult to interpret. A U.S. Food and Drug Administration (FDA) Advisory Panel concluded that there was insufficient evidence to conclude that rasagiline has disease-slowing properties. What confounded these outcomes (as well as some of the earlier trials) was that the study drug also had symptomatic benefits (i.e., treated Parkinson's disease symptoms). Since the outcome measures were clinical assessments of parkinsonism, it was difficult to distinguish symptomatic benefit from slowed disease progression.

Other drugs that have been studied as potential agents to slow the progression of Parkinson's disease include creatine (used by muscle builders) and the antibiotic minocycline. To date, no proof has been produced showing that these or any other agents truly have a disease-slowing benefit.

WHAT ABOUT COENZYME Q10?

Mitochondria are components of all human and animal cells and are responsible for the ultimate conversion of food products into usable cellular energy. They are the cellular location for aerobic metabolism, where oxygen interacts with biochemically processed sugars, fats, and proteins to generate high-energy molecules. These high-energy molecules (primarily adenosine triphosphate [ATP]) are crucial factors driving a vast array of important biochemical reactions in both humans and animals. Numerous studies have documented reduced mitochondrial function in people with Parkinson's disease. Investigators have speculated that mitochondrial dysfunction might be a contributory factor in, or at least a clue to, the cause of Parkinson's disease.

Coenzyme Q10 is a cofactor in one important component of mitochondrial function. Coenzyme Q10 can be purchased as a synthetic supplement from health food stores and taken by mouth. Approximately a decade ago, a small randomized clinical trial assessed orally administered coenzyme Q10 as a possible disease-slowing drug among patients with Parkinson's disease. Compared to the group given placebo pills, the group administered the largest coenzyme Q10 dosage, 1200 mg daily, performed significantly better than the placebo group when assessed after approximately 1.5 years of treatment. However, the two other groups administered lower coenzyme Q10 dosages (300 mg or 600 mg daily) did no better than the placebo group. The investigators acknowledged that with the small numbers of patients in this particular study the finding needed replication in larger studies. Unfortunately, two subsequent studies funded by the National Institute of Health failed to replicate this benefit, despite larger coenzyme Q10 dosages (and many more patients). The current consensus among neurologists is that evidence does not support administration of coenzyme Q10 for Parkinson's disease. By inference its effect should be no different for DLB.

LIVING LONGER WITH LEVODOPA

The prototypic Lewy disorder, Parkinson's disease, has been treated with levodopa pills since it was approved by the FDA about 40 years ago. As we will discuss in later chapters, levodopa is a natural substance. It is normally present in our bodies and in our diets. It is from a class of natural compounds called amino acids, which are the building blocks of proteins. Proteins in our body and in our diet consist of strings of amino acids.

Soon after levodopa became available, eight different investigative teams analyzed longevity among patients with Parkinson's disease, comparing mortality rates from the period just before to that just after levodopa availability. All eight published reports documented substantially longer lifespans for patients with Parkinson's disease that coincided with the advent of levodopa.

If levodopa treatment for Parkinson's disease results in longer lifespans, what is the underlying mechanism? Intuitively, it seems most likely that this outcome reflects the substantially improved mobility that accompanies levodopa treatment of Parkinson's disease. Prior to its availability, untreated Parkinson's disease patients became progressively immobile, sedentary, and eventually chair- or bed-bound. Such an immobile existence predisposes to major general health risks, such as blood clots in the legs or aspiration pneumonias. Likely, improved longevity relates to keeping patients mobile and active, rather than to some specific biochemical effect on the cause of Parkinson's disease.

Perhaps this lesson still needs to be taught: sedentary lifestyles and lack of physical activity may be detrimental to one's health. The human body may indeed obey the rule "if you don't use it, you lose it."

EXERCISE AS A POSSIBLE DISEASE-SLOWING STRATEGY

Whereas drugs have failed to slow the progression of Lewy disorders, simple aerobic exercise may be effective. Intuitively, it makes sense that physical activity would keep the muscles toned and would counter deconditioning. Beyond that, however, there is now a large amount of compelling medical and scientific literature arguing that aerobic exercise may slow brain aging and reduce later risks of cognitive impairment or dementia. Moreover, exercise may stabilize or improve cognition that has already been compromised by neurodegenerative disease.

These findings have been documented in humans, and the basis for these findings has been studied in animal experiments.

Animal studies have documented remarkable benefits of exercise in facilitating maintenance and new development of brain (synaptic) connections. Exercised animals generate brain neurotrophic factors; such neurotrophic factors are natural substances that favor brain health and development, much like fertilizer on a lawn. Compared to sedentary animals, exercised animals have not only biochemical but also microscopic and electrophysiologic evidence of facilitated brain neuroplasticity, that is, brain circuit connectivity. The evidence for a neuroprotective effect with aerobic exercise is presented in Chapter 20.

The implications from this evidence favoring aerobic exercise to counter neurodegeneration and aging are two-fold. First, an active exercise routine may be neuroprotective. Second, for DLB patients with parkinsonian features, it is crucial that the physician provide adequate levodopa coverage to enable physical activities. As we will discuss in later chapters, parkinsonism is a component of not only Parkinson's disease but also DLB; levodopa therapy potentially improves mobility and the capacity to be active in both conditions.

4

Symptoms, Related Brain Regions, and Diagnosis

As a prelude to the treatment chapters that follow, we need to define and describe the types of problems and symptoms encountered in DLB and PDD. The clinical picture can be quite varied: problems encountered by one person may be quite different from those encountered by another person, and symptoms that are problematic in one individual may be minimal in another.

In these disorders, the Lewy neurodegenerative process potentially affects certain nervous system regions but spares others. Affected areas include thinking and memory circuits, as well as movement (motor) function and the autonomic nervous system, which regulates primary functions such as bladder, bowel, and blood pressure control. Many other brain regions, by contrast, are spared or minimally involved, such as vision and sensation.

BACKGROUND: CENTRAL NERVOUS SYSTEM ORGANIZATION, FROM CORTEX TO SPINAL CORD

The brain and spinal cord constitute the central nervous system. The interface between the brain and spinal cord is by way of

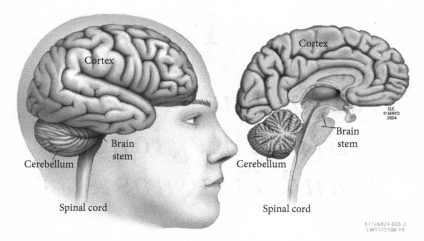

Figure 4.1 Illustration of brain depicting connections with the spinal cord and illustrating cortex.

the brain stem, as shown in Figure 4.1. Thought, memory, and reasoning are primarily organized in the thick layers of cortex overlying lower brain levels.

Volitional movements, such as writing, throwing, or kicking, also emanate from the cortex and integrate with circuits just below, including those in the basal ganglia, shown in Figure 4.2. The basal ganglia includes the striatum, globus pallidus, subthalamic nucleus, and substantia nigra, as illustrated in Figure 4.2. Movement information is integrated and modulated in these basal ganglia nuclei and then transmitted down the brain stem to the spinal cord. At spinal cord levels the correct sequence of muscle activation that has been programmed is accomplished. Activated nerves from appropriate regions of the spinal cord relay the signals to the proper muscles. Sensory information from the periphery (limbs) travels in the opposite direction.

How are these signals transmitted? Brain cells called neurons have long, wire-like extensions that interface with other neurons, effectively making up circuits that are slightly similar to computer circuits; this is illustrated in Figure 4.3. At the end of these wire-like extensions are tiny enlargements (terminals) that

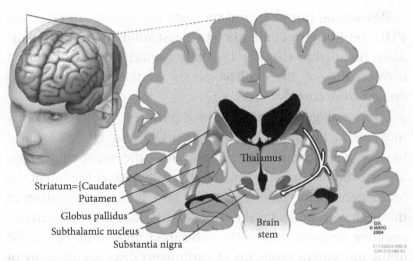

Figure 4.2   Brain slice revealing basal ganglia regions, including the substantia nigra and striatum.

contain specific biological chemicals called neurotransmitters. Neurotransmitters are released when the electrical signal travels down that neuron to the end of that wire-like process. It is the release of a particular neurotransmitter that activates or inhibits the next neuron in the circuit.

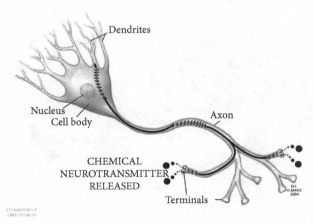

Figure 4.3   Prototypic neuron, the fundamental cell of the nervous system.

Reasoning, thinking, and memory are affected in DLB and PDD, resulting in dementia or at least mild cognitive impairment (defined in Chapter 1). These cognitive problems reflect involvement of the highest levels of the central nervous system—the cortex (Figure 4.1).

The basal ganglia, shown in Figure 4.2, modulates body movement, including walking. In PDD and DLB, a crucial basal ganglia component degenerates—the substantia nigra. The substantia nigra is located in the midbrain at the top of the brain stem, depicted in Figure 4.4. The dark pigmentation of this region accounts for the name of this nucleus. The relatively selective degeneration of the substantia nigra underlies most of the movement problems of Parkinson's disease and many of those in DLB and PDD.

As stated earlier, neurons signal other neurons via release of tiny amounts of specific biological chemicals, or neurotransmitters (Figure 4.3). The substantia nigra uses the neurotransmitter dopamine for such signaling; in fact, it floods the next link in the brain circuit with dopamine, the striatum (Figure 4.2). Dopamine is a neurotransmitter not found in many other brain circuits, and when the substantia nigra is lost, brain concentrations of dopamine plummet. With this decline of dopamine in

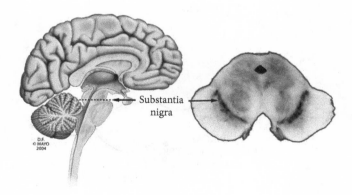

Figure 4.4 The substantia nigra is located at the top of the brain stem (midbrain).

the striatum, movement is slowed and the amplitude of movement diminished. This is termed "parkinsonism," implying the appearance of Parkinson's disease.

THE AUTONOMIC NERVOUS SYSTEM

The autonomic nervous system is connected to the brain and spinal cord but works somewhat independently and automatically. Most of what is programmed and organized by the autonomic nervous system is unconscious and largely reflexive. These functions include control of bladder, bowels, blood pressure, and sweating, as depicted in Figure 4.5.

Consider bladder function. The kidneys generate urine that passes down a conduit (ureter) to the bladder, as shown in Figure 4.6. When the bladder nears full capacity, a reflex is triggered that brings this to conscious awareness, resulting in the

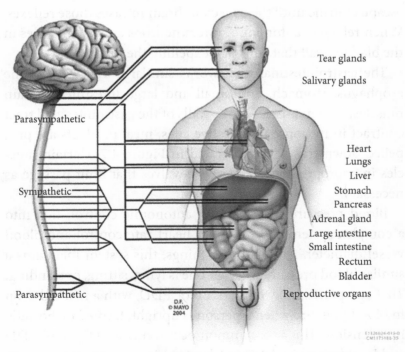

Figure 4.5 The components of the autonomic nervous system.

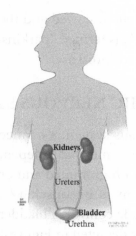

Figure 4.6 The urinary system. The kidneys generate the urine, which is collected in the bladder, a reservoir. The conduits from the kidneys to bladder are the ureters. Urine is expelled via the urethra.

urge to urinate. However, internal bladder reflexes prevent the escape of urine until the conscious brain releases those reflexes. When released, autonomic system neurons activate muscles in the bladder wall that contract, expelling the urine.

The gastrointestinal tract works similarly. The walls of the esophagus, stomach, and small and large intestines contain muscles. When muscles in the walls of the gastrointestinal tract contract in response to digestive cues, meal products are propelled downstream, as illustrated in Figure 4.7. Certain muscles in appropriate places serve as valves that limit passage as necessary.

Blood pressure is also under autonomic control, tied into a complex system and linked to heart rate control and blood vessel diameter. Among other things, this system maintains a similar blood pressure whether one is lying, sitting, or standing. That component may fail in DLB or PDD, with a marked drop in blood pressure when a person is upright, termed orthostatic hypotension. This is a common occurrence in DLB and PDD and is addressed in detail in Chapter 13.

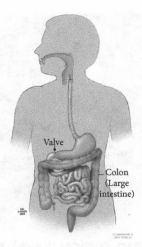

Valve

Colon
(Large
intestine)

Figure 4.7 The digestive tract, from mouth to anus.

WHAT IS AFFECTED IN LEWY CONDITIONS?

DLB and PDD affect combinations of various nervous system circuits. Symptoms include impairment of cognition (including thinking and memory), movement (parkinsonism), autonomic control (bladder, bowel, blood pressure), and sleep, as well as psychiatric problems. Let us consider the character of each of these disorders in detail before focusing on treatment in subsequent chapters.

COGNITIVE PROFILE OF DLB AND PDD

Thinking, memory, judgment, reasoning, and organizational skills are affected in DLB and PDD. The substrate for these problems is predominantly the cortex, shown in Figure 4.1. The cortex is the thick mantle of cognitive and other high-level circuits overlying lower brain regions. Specific cortical regions mediate different aspects of perception, cognitive processing, and intellect. These regions include the frontal, parietal, temporal, and occipital lobes, shown in Figure 4.8.

The cognitive profile of DLB is distinctive and differs from that of Alzheimer's disease. Alzheimer's disease especially affects

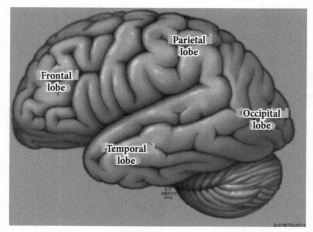

Figure 4.8 The primary cortices (lobes) of the brain.

memory and learning, as well as language. These are typically less affected in DLB, in contrast to other cognitive areas. The temporal lobe (Figure 4.8), where memory and language circuits are concentrated, appears to be an early target of Alzheimer's disease.

DLB and PDD tend to affect other cortical regions more prominently, as reflected in the cognitive symptoms. Two components of intellect that are often impaired in DLB and PDD are executive function and visuospatial conceptualization.

Executive Function

Executive skills are mediated by the frontal cortex (frontal lobe, shown in Figure 4.8). Problems with executive functioning can be quite variable but may include one or more deficiencies in the following areas:

- Organizing, planning, preparing for future events
- Responding to complex or novel tasks or surroundings
- Mental flexibility or concept formation
- Shifting attention, or mental focusing
- Multitasking

Thus, the executive frontal lobe allows us to focus on issues or projects at hand, yet shift attention when that becomes important.

When we are engaged in more than one activity, it permits us to not only multitask but also specifically attend to one task when that takes on paramount importance. The frontal lobe mediates cognitive flexibility yet keeps the focus on-target when appropriate. Importantly, it is also responsible for organizing and triggering appropriate social responses and interactions. The frontal lobe executive dysfunction in DLB or PDD may manifest as poor judgment, lack of common sense, poor planning, or failure to prioritize. It may lead to "brain-lock" when an affected individual starts some simple task, not knowing how to start or how to organize the activity. Similarly, it may result in doing less important things first or in an inappropriate order. These difficulties may translate into projects taking twice as long to complete.

Social interactions may also be compromised when the frontal lobes are affected. Those with DLB or PDD may be slower to pick up on nonverbal cues, such as facial gestures, body language, or voice intonation. This reaction may compromise communication and can impair spousal interactions. Previously laid-back and thoughtful individuals may become impatient and impulsive. Spouses are often the first to recognize such subtle changes in personality.

On the other hand, some people with DLB or PDD can become apathetic; this is probably also of frontal cortex origin. Previously highly functioning people with busy schedules become couch potatoes. Sometimes this is recognized by the patient and is a major complaint to the physician. For others, it is only the spouse and family who recognize the change in behavior.

Decline in judgment may be coupled with impulsivity in those with frontal lobe problems, resulting in poor decision-making. Thus, business and investment decisions may require scrutiny from another family member.

Visuospatial Function

Problems perceiving and conceptualizing in two- and three-dimensional space are also typical of DLB and PDD. This may appear as difficulty reading a map or interpreting complex pictures, or getting lost in a familiar neighborhood. Blueprints, roadmaps, and housing floor patterns become less interpretable to those with DLB or PDD. Visuospatial disorders may be detected in the clinic by having the person draw a clock or copy a cube. The clock drawn may not have all the numbers apportioned in the correct places, with large gaps in some clock regions. The three dimensions of a cube may not be perceived when the person is trying to copy this figure, generating a two-dimensional drawn box.

Visuospatial perception and conception tends to be localized in the parietal cortex and regions connected to it. Just behind the parietal cortex is the primary visual area of the brain, the occipital cortex (Figure 4.8). These elementary vision circuits in the occipital lobe are linked to parietal circuits integrating what we see with what we conceptualize.

Memory

Memory is affected in DLB and PDD, but not as severely as in Alzheimer's disease, where memory loss is typically the earliest problem. Correspondingly, the temporal lobes, where memories are encoded (Figure 4.8), are much less affected in DLB and PDD than in Alzheimer's disease. In Alzheimer's disease, names of familiar friends, important appointments, and conversations are quickly forgotten. As Alzheimer's disease progresses, events just a few minutes before may not be recalled, despite prompting or providing clues. In contrast, those with DLB or PDD who forget things may be helped by a reminder or a cue. Those with Lewy disorders may forget names but will often be able to select the correct name from a list.

In DLB and PDD, lack of attention or poor mental organization may contribute to memory impairment. This aspect is attributable to frontal lobe dysfunction (Figure 4.8). Most of us can remember a list of items better if organized into groups.

For example, a grocery list of "sausage, hamburger, lettuce, and cucumber" is easier to recall if lumped into two groups such as "meats" and "produce." In Lewy disorders, such mental organization may not readily occur. Problems along these lines may impair the ability to organize and execute all but the simplest medication regimens, and this can be problematic for older adults with long medication lists.

Fluctuations in Thinking and Alertness

Unique to these Lewy dementias is the fluctuation of mental clarity. People with DLB or PDD may be alert and lucid during portions of the day, but inexplicably confused several hours later. This is a hallmark of DLB and PDD. Daytime drowsiness may similarly fluctuate like this, although there may be other treatable reasons for sleepiness, as discussed in Chapters 9 and 16. The reason for these fluctuations in mental clarity is unknown.

Hallucinations and Delusions

Uncommon in Alzheimer's disease but common in DLB and PDD are hallucinations and delusions, defined as follows.

Hallucinations

Seeing things that are not there and hearing voices are two different types of hallucinations. In DLB and PDD, hallucinations are almost exclusively visual, characterized by seeing illusory people in the house or strangers walking in the yard. Although certain medications may exacerbate or provoke these, they often occur in the absence of any such drugs.

Delusions

Delusions are false beliefs, such as paranoid thinking, or bizarre imaginings, such as concerns that the spouse is having an affair.

PARKINSONISM OF DLB AND PDD

Parkinsonism implies movement problems that resemble those of Parkinson's disease. This is obviously expected in Parkinson's disease advancing to dementia (PDD). However, the same problems occur in DLB, albeit to variable degrees. The primary mechanism for this parkinsonism is degeneration of the substantia nigra. As stated earlier, the substantia nigra floods the striatum with dopamine, which is crucial to the functioning of that brain region (Figure 4.2). Fortunately, the low levels of striatal dopamine can be replenished with levodopa therapy, as addressed in detail in Chapters 5–8. Hence the walking and movement problems encountered in these disorders may be quite treatable.

Classic parkinsonian movement symptoms include the following:

- *Resting tremor, typically of the hands, but often of the foot or leg and sometimes chin*
  A *resting tremor* implies that the limb (or chin) is not being voluntarily activated but rather is in a resting or relaxed position. Tremor may be absent in approximately 20% of those with Parkinson's disease. This PD resting tremor differs from a more common condition, *essential tremor*, where the tremor is only present when the limb (hand) is being used (i.e., not at rest). Essential tremor may also include head or voice tremor, which are not components of Parkinson's disease.
- *Slowness of movement, known as bradykinesia*
  Not only are movements slowed but the amplitude of movements is also reduced; this is what gives handwriting the classic "micrographic" appearance (smaller size due to reduced amplitude of the repetitive hand movements when writing).
- *Stiffness of the limbs or neck, termed rigidity*
  Rigidity is not just the stiffness of aging or the joint problems of arthritis but rather increased muscle tone in a limb, causing resistance when an examiner moves a "relaxed" limb.

- *Walking problems, such as shortened stride-length, shuffling gait, and sometimes imbalance*
  Accompanying such problems is reduced swing of the arm(s) and often a stooped posture.
- *Loss of automatic movements*
  Many of our actions are normally done outside of conscious awareness and tend to be lost or attenuated in these Lewy disorders. There may be reduced eye blinking, loss of arm swing when walking, and diminished gesturing when talking. The classic "masked face" of parkinsonism is also an example of this.

In these Lewy conditions the problems are typically asymmetric, affecting one side of the body more than the other. In fact, during the early years, they may be confined to one side of the body.

Although dopamine deficiency from the degeneration of the substantia nigra is responsible for many or even most of these problems, other basal ganglia regions become affected in advanced disease. Since these additionally affected brain regions do not use dopamine as a neurotransmitter, levodopa and related drugs do not help.

DYSAUTONOMIA IN PDD AND DLB

Autonomic nervous system involvement may translate into the following:

- Impaired bladder function, including urinary urgency (sudden need to urinate), incontinence, or slowed emptying
- Slowed transit of meals out of the stomach and into the small intestine (delayed gastric emptying), often with bloating and a feeling of fullness
- Constipation
- Orthostatic hypotension, which is a drop in blood pressure when a person is upright (resulting in faintness or actual fainting when standing or walking)
- Reduced perspiration (usually unrecognized)
- Erectile dysfunction in men

Microscopic Lewy neurodegenerative changes may be found throughout the autonomic nervous system.

SLEEP DISORDERS IN DLB AND PDD

A variety of sleep disorders occur in DLB, Parkinson's disease, and PDD and are summarized below.

REM Sleep Behavior Disorder

Normally when we dream while asleep our bodies are limp, preventing movement during vivid dreams. Only our eyes are active during this sleep stage, called rapid eye movement sleep (REM). In people with REM sleep behavior, the body does not go limp when dreaming (termed, dream enactment behavior). Such individuals talk, kick, punch, or act out in other ways as they are asleep and dreaming. This is a primary symptom of DLB, PDD, and Parkinson's disease. It may precede other symptoms of these disorders by years or even decades. The cause is thought to relate to degeneration of a small brain stem region. This disorder is treatable and addressed in Chapter 17.

Insomnia

Insomnia is common among humans. However, it is much more frequent among those with DLB, PDD, and Parkinson's disease. Often it relates to the discomfort of inadequately replenished brain dopamine with consequent restlessness and stiffness. This cause of insomnia is treatable with dopamine replenishment (Chapter 9).

Daytime Drowsiness

Sleepiness during the daytime is common in DLB and PDD and has a variety of possible causes:

- Poor night-time sleep
- Disturbed breathing during sleep (sleep apnea)

- Repetitive jerking during sleep (periodic leg movements of sleep)
- Prescription medications

These are treatable conditions and are addressed in detail in Chapter 16.

Disturbed Sleep Architecture

Impaired sleep cycles may also be a primary symptom of DLB or PDD. This may manifest as prolonged sleep or occasionally mid-day deep-sleep from which the sleeper cannot be easily aroused.

PSYCHIATRIC SYMPTOMS IN DLB AND PDD

Psychiatric issues are common but often treatable. They include anxiety, depression, hallucinations and delusions. These do not necessarily correlate with cognitive or movement problems. For most of these symptoms, the precise region of the brain that is responsible is unknown.

Depression

Having DLB or PDD might make anyone depressed. However, depression in these conditions may have a basis in Lewy degeneration of the dopamine or of certain other neurotransmitter systems, such as serotonin or norepinephrine neurons. These neurotransmitters can be replenished through medications, as discussed later in Chapter 18.

Anxiety

Nervousness, anxiety, and restlessness are all common in DLB, PDD, and Parkinson's disease. In many cases, these symptoms respond to adequate replenishment of brain dopamine with carbidopa/levodopa; hence the nigrostriatal system is implicated (see Chapter 9).

Hallucinations (Visual)

Seeing illusory people, animals, or objects while wide awake is common in both DLB and PDD. These are different from vivid dreams, which occur during sleep. Although hallucinations may be provoked by certain medications, they also occur as a direct result of the Lewy disorder. These are treatable, as detailed in Chapter 10.

Delusions

Nonsensical beliefs with no basis in reality unfortunately develop in a small group of people with DLB or PDD. While certain medications may facilitate this problem, it is primarily due to the underlying disease process. Examples include paranoia or irrational concerns about marital affairs. Another example is Capgras syndrome, in which a spouse or family member is not recognized and thought to be an impostor. Like hallucinations, these can be treated (Chapter 10).

Apathy

Apathy implies a loss of motivation, interest, and energy, which appears to be a fundamental component of Lewy conditions in some people. The basal ganglia is one of the crucial areas of the brain responsible for motivation, and dopamine deficiency may contribute to apathy. Depression or poor sleep may also play a role. Apathy can be difficult to treat but may respond to medications directed at each of the potential contributors: depression, basal ganglia dopamine deficiency, or impaired sleep.

THE DIAGNOSES

How is the Diagnosis of DLB Made?

The diagnosis of dementia with Lewy bodies is not made on the basis of a brain imaging study or laboratory test. The diagnosis is primarily based on clinical findings obtained during the clinician's assessment. This includes two components: the history and the neurologic examination.

The history is what the patient, spouse, partner, or family tells the clinician. When did this problem begin? Did it start suddenly? Was it associated with other symptoms, such as fever, headache? Those individuals who are quite demented may not be of much help in this regard and a collateral history from someone who knows the person well is crucial.

The neurologic examination is done in the clinician's office and involves assessment of walking, coordination, and reflexes. If parkinsonism is present it will be detected on this examination. While limited tests of cognition may be done as part of this office visit, a more comprehensive cognitive examination by a psychologist may be scheduled. This separate psychometric testing will assess not only severity of thinking impairment but also the cognitive profile, including various aspects of intellectual function such as executive function, visuospatial abilities, and memory.

Beyond this, testing is done to exclude other causes or contributing factors. As detailed in Chapter 12, when confronted with a demented person, clinicians must consider all factors capable of impairing brain function. Brain imaging is typically done to look for evidence of some other cause, such as a tumor, stroke, or hemorrhage. This might include brain magnetic resonance imaging (MRI) or computed tomography (CT). Blood work is done because confusion has a myriad of general causes or contributors such as liver or kidney failure, thyroid problems, or vitamin B12 deficiency. Specific components of Lewy body disease may be investigated further with testing, such as autonomic or sleep studies.

Brain imaging to detect brain dopamine deficiency is available, but usually it is unnecessary, except for research purposes. This involves administration of a drug that selectively concentrates in the dopamine system of the striatum; a radioactive marker is attached to the drug, giving off a radioactive signal that is detected by the scanning device. Dopamine deficiencies due to Lewy disorders are associated with markedly reduced signals of this type from the striatum.

The clinician suspecting DLB needs to consider the composite of symptoms discussed in this chapter. If no other cause is identified (e.g., strokes, blood disorder), then the findings on the history and examination are the primary factors used in establishing the diagnosis, although psychometric (cognitive), autonomic, and sleep test results may provide valuable clues.

People with DLB are quite different from one another. In some, the parkinsonism may be the paramount problem, whereas in others it may be the dementia or even the autonomic problems. In other words, the various symptoms summarized in this chapter can be put together into every conceivable combination. Hence, the clinician must think broadly; there is no one specific prototypic DLB presentation that fits everyone.

Investigators have tried to formalize the diagnostic process, and a consensus panel has established diagnostic criteria, under the auspices of Professor Ian McKeith from the United Kingdom. Rather than provide their extensive and complicated algorithm, let us instead put ourselves in the mind of the doctor in the clinic assessing someone suspected of having DLB. We will assume that the dementia workup has detected no other cause, and that treatable causes have been excluded. We are left with the task of attaching a name to a neurodegenerative condition that includes dementia. The composite of the symptoms and the examination findings are the basis for the diagnosis; these may include combinations of what was detailed in earlier portions of this chapter:

- Cognitive impairment, especially with the profile discussed above that includes executive and visuospatial dysfunction, although memory loss is a typical part of this
- Visual hallucinations or delusions
- Parkinsonism, typically responsive to carbidopa/levodopa

- Autonomic problems: bladder control difficulties, constipation, or orthostatic hypotension
- Sleep disorder that especially includes REM sleep behavior disorder
- Marked fluctuations in mental clarity (occasionally)

By virtue of the McKeith criteria, the parkinsonism should not have preceded the dementia by more than a year. If it did, Parkinson's disease with dementia (PDD) would be diagnosed, which is discussed next.

How Is PDD Diagnosed?

DLB can be difficult to diagnose, especially early in the disease course when some of the typical symptoms have not yet become fully manifest. In contrast, PDD is a relatively straightforward diagnosis. PDD obviously starts as simple Parkinson's disease; however, over years, some patients with Parkinson's disease develop dementia. The likelihood of dementia relates especially to age and the duration of Parkinson's disease: the longer a person has Parkinson's disease and the older they are, the greater the risk of dementia.

The clinician making the diagnosis of PDD must exclude other causes of cognitive impairment (see Chapter 12). If they are excluded, then what else could it be? The only complexity is the McKeith 1-year rule, cited earlier. To qualify as PDD, rather than DLB, the parkinsonism must have been present for more than a year before the cognitive symptoms developed. Obviously, this is a little arbitrary, but such distinctions help researchers clearly define what they are studying. In the clinic, where clinicians deal with real people and their problems, that distinction is less crucial.

HOW TO USE THE TREATMENT PORTION OF THIS BOOK

The chapters that follow are divided into individual problems that develop to differing extents among people with DLB or

PDD. They can be read out of order, depending on the reader's needs. The organization allows these issues to be addressed individually, with topics broken down as follows:

- Levodopa-responsive problems: parkinsonism, anxiety, pain, insomnia
- Problems exacerbated by Parkinson's medications: hallucinations, delusions, pathologic behaviors
- Cognitive problems
- Dysautonomia, including orthostatic hypotension and bladder and bowel problems
- Sleep problems: drowsiness, insomnia, dream enactment behavior
- More general issues that relate to general medical problems, exercise, hospitalizations, caregivers, and patient living arrangements

The focus in all subsequent chapters will be on practical treatment strategies.

TREATMENT

The chapters that follow are the meat of the book and are subdivided according to specific problems. People with DLB or PDD do not necessarily experience all of these difficulties; they may be absent or only of modest consequence.

These chapters do not need to be read in their entirety, but it would be wise to at least skim them all. If something surfaces in the future, knowing where to look will be helpful.

Certain problems respond well to the medication used to treat simple Parkinson's disease, carbidopa/levodopa. This medication replenishes a neurotransmitter, dopamine, that is deficient in the brains of not only those with Parkinson's disease but also DLB. (Neurotransmitters are substances used by brain cells [neurons] for signaling the next neuron in a brain circuit.) We will address these levodopa-responsive problems first, and then conditions requiring drugs from other classes.

As a prelude to these treatment chapters, a few comments, based on clinical experience, are worth noting:

1. Sometimes fewer rather than more medications are preferable.
2. Newer drugs are sometimes not as good as some of the older drugs.
3. Commercial (monied) interests may skew the treatment advice.
4. Treatment of one problem may upset the apple cart in another area (unintended consequences).

A little knowledge plus common sense will go a long way toward optimizing treatment of DLB and PDD.

LEVODOPA-RESPONSIVE

PROBLEMS

Some of the more troublesome symptoms of DLB, PDD, and Parkinson's disease are due to loss of the brain neurotransmitter dopamine. Dopamine is crucial for movement; without it movements slow or are stalled and tremor may occur.

Dopamine taken in pill form cannot get into the brain. However, the natural precursor of dopamine, levodopa, does get into the brain and is rapidly transformed into dopamine. The discovery in the 1960s that low brain dopamine was responsible for many of the symptoms of Parkinson's disease was revolutionary; it markedly transformed the lives of people with Parkinson's disease. A similar dopamine deficiency state is typically present in people with DLB and lends itself to levodopa treatment. The next five chapters focus on problems that can be treated with levodopa therapy.

The primary target of levodopa is the movement problems that characterize parkinsonism. Several chapters are devoted to defining parkinsonism, as well as the rationale for certain medication strategies and how to initiate and adjust drug doses. Chapter 9 addresses non-movement problems that reflect dopamine deficiency and benefit from levodopa therapy, most notably anxiety and insomnia.

5

Which Drug for Parkinsonism?

Walking, Stiffness, Tremor, and Slowness

In Chapters 1 and 4, we briefly summarized the symptoms of parkinsonism. Parkinsonism implies movement problems that are typical of Parkinson's disease. They remain treatment issues during the lifetime of people with Parkinson's disease, even if dementia develops. Similarly, parkinsonism also typically occurs in DLB, although to variable degrees. In these disorders parkinsonism primarily reflects low brain dopamine levels and improves with dopamine replacement therapy, often markedly.

HOW IS PARKINSONISM DETERMINED?

Parkinsonism occurs when a region of the brain called the basal ganglia ceases to work properly (see Figure 4.2 in Chapter 4). As discussed in Chapter 4, the substantia nigra is a crucial regulator of basal ganglia activity, which is mediated by dopamine release in the striatum. The substantia nigra degenerates in these Lewy disorders and, as a result, brain dopamine declines. With a decline in dopamine, movement slows. *Bradykinesia* is the medical term for such slowness. This manifests as not only slowed movement but also less movement and smaller than normal movements. Unconscious automatic movements, such as blinking or arm swing, diminish. A unique tremor of the hands (sometimes legs) often develops when these limbs are in a relaxed position (rest tremor). For unknown reasons, the brain is not affected symmetrically, hence, neither is the body. Typically, one side of the body is much more impaired than the other.

The extent to which these symptoms develop differs from person to person and includes various combinations of the following components.

Bradykinesia

The slowness may be apparent on one or both sides of the body. For example, one leg may lag behind when walking. The overall appearance is characterized by moving much slower than expected for one's age. The person feels as if they are moving in molasses—everything slows down.

Impaired Repetitive Movements

Many of our daily activities involve repeated small movements, such as writing or brushing teeth. In the Lewy conditions of DLB and PDD, the size (amplitude) of repetitive movements diminishes, impairing the activity. This is exemplified by the small handwriting of someone with parkinsonism, termed micrographia.

Clinicians assess repetitive motor function by asking the patient to repetitively tap the thumb and index finger. With parkinsonism, these movements tend to slow and the movements become smaller. Correspondingly, fine motor tasks, such as buttoning, become harder.

Loss of Automatic Movements

People normally move spontaneously and unconsciously, such as blinking their eyes, swinging their arms while walking, or gesturing when talking; facial animation similarly occurs without thinking about it. With parkinsonism, these automatic movements tend to diminish. This is exemplified in the "masked face" of parkinsonism, where eye blinking declines and the face no longer displays much emotion. Sometimes this is misinterpreted as appearing depressed.

Rigidity

The stiffness of parkinsonism (rigidity) is due to increased muscle tension across joints. It is often more prominent on one side of the body (asymmetric) and may be accompanied by pain from this muscle tension state. Doctors assess rigidity by slowly moving the person's elbow or knee while the person tries to relax. Involuntary resistance to that movement constitutes rigidity.

Gait Problems

Walking is affected in a variety of ways. First, walking may be slower (bradykinesia), and walking partners will often note an inability of the person with parkinsonism to keep up. Second, the stride length diminishes and steps shorten. Third, the striding foot may no longer land on the heel but rather flat on the sole. This is in contrast to the normal stride, in which one lands on the heel and pushes off the ball of the foot. With shortened stride length and loss of the heel strike, the gait may have a "shuffling" appearance. In addition, turning can be problematic, requiring multiple small steps instead of using a smooth pivot.

Superimposed on this may be "freezing" of gait. This implies that the feet are stuck to the floor, as if held by a magnet. This characteristically occurs when the affected person starts to walk, turn, or go through doorways. Interestingly, once walking starts, the gait may become normal until the person stops or turns.

Stooped Posture

Normally, our posture is controlled by the brain, which adjusts the tone of the longitudinally running muscles along our spinal column. Too much tone in one direction will pull the trunk that way. That is exactly what tends to happen in parkinsonism, resulting in a stooped posture. (It also tends to occur to mild degrees with normal aging.) Sometimes this process disproportionately affects the neck, pulling it in one direction. Most of the time, however, the trunk is simply pulled forward.

Imbalance

Imbalance is common in Lewy disorders, but often it does not translate into a major fall risk until either later ages (beyond age 75 to 80 years) or there is long-standing disease. Clinicians may assess balance problems by the "pull test." Here, the examiner stands behind the patient and then pulls back on both of the person's shoulders. Normal people easily resist this backward pull by extending their upper trunk backward or taking a step back. Those with parkinsonian imbalance may "retropulse" backward into the examiner's arms. Unfortunately, unlike other aspects of parkinsonism, poor balance rarely responds to dopamine replacement therapy.

Rest Tremor

The majority of tremor conditions seen in neurology clinics do not represent Parkinson's disease or DLB. Classic Lewy tremor is manifest when the limb is not being activated, that is, it is "at rest." Characteristically, a tremulous hand (or fingers) is apparent when the hand is resting in the lap or at one's side when walking. Similarly, a lower limb resting tremor may be seen when the person is seated with the leg resting on the floor. A rest tremor of the hand (or leg) sometimes persists when that limb is held in an extended posture; however, it typically stops during movement.

Essential tremor is a much more common tremor condition that should not be confused with the rest tremor of Lewy disorders. In essential tremor, a hand tremor is rarely present in the resting position but develops when the hand is activated, such as when using an eating utensil or when writing. Head tremor or voice tremor is never a Lewy tremor but rather is typical of essential tremor.

Hypophonia and Hypokinetic Dysarthria

Hypophonia refers to the softer voice of Lewy conditions. Typically associated with this is less precise enunciation, termed hypokinetic dysarthria. This is due to the same movement problems that affect the hands during repetitive tasks, but in this case the lips, tongue, and palate are affected.

Other Parkinsonian Issues

Difficulty rising from the seated position is common in parkinsonism, despite normal lower limb strength. Swallowing may be affected, although usually not severely. There are also a number of other symptoms that do not involve movement or motor function, such as anxiety, depression, insomnia, and even pain. These are common in Parkinson's disease and are termed non-motor symptoms; they similarly occur in DLB and PDD.

Combinations of any of the symptoms described in this section constitute parkinsonism. They are expected to improve with dopamine replacement therapy, specifically with levodopa. The only exception is prominent imbalance—dopamine does not appear to be the neurotransmitter involved in balance systems.

WHO SHOULD BE TREATED WITH A DOPAMINE REPLACEMENT MEDICATION?

The goals for treating parkinsonism in the context of DLB or PDD vary with age, disability, and other medical issues. In general, if walking or other aspects of life are impaired by parkinsonism, then an oral dopamine replacement medication (e.g., levodopa) should be considered. Alternatively, if parkinsonism is making a minimal contribution to disability, this can be deferred.

For some people more limited goals may be appropriate. For example, those with an advanced medical condition or major orthopedic problems may have difficulty returning to an ambulatory state. Major imbalance also does not reverse with medications. While return to walking ability may not be possible for some individuals, levodopa treatment may facilitate self-hygiene or bed-to-chair transfers, providing assistance to caregivers.

As discussed in Chapter 20, exercise is important for maintaining not only general health but also brain health. If exercise capability can be facilitated by dopamine replacement (i.e., levodopa), that is an appropriate goal.

WHICH DRUG FOR DOPAMINE REPLACEMENT?

The drugs primarily used to treat parkinsonism target brain dopamine, either by increasing it or by acting like dopamine. There are four primary classes of drugs used for this purpose, as follows.

Levodopa

This is the natural dopamine precursor, which everyone has in their body. It is one biochemical step removed from dopamine. When administered in pill form, an enzyme present throughout the body is able to convert it to dopamine. Although dopamine per se cannot cross into the brain, levodopa is transported across the natural barrier between the bloodstream and brain (blood–brain barrier).

In pill form, levodopa is combined with carbidopa, which prevents it from being prematurely metabolized outside the brain. Hence, the standard formulation in the United States is carbidopa/levodopa (Sinemet). (In this text, brand names of drugs are capitalized and listed between parentheses after the generic form.) Carbidopa is crucial for reducing nausea. Outside the United States, benserazide is often used instead of carbidopa, but the effects are essentially identical.

Dopamine Agonists

Dopamine agonists chemically resemble dopamine but do not provide the full spectrum of benefit that occurs with natural dopamine. The two pill forms are ropinirole (Requip) and pramipexole (Mirapex). A patch containing the dopamine agonist rotigotine (Neupro) is also available.

Inhibitors of the Brain Monoamine Oxidase-B (MAO-B)

MAO is a dopamine-degrading enzyme found within the brain and elsewhere. Blocking the B-form of this enzyme mildly increases brain dopamine concentrations. The two available drugs from this class are rasagiline (Azilect) and selegiline (Eldepryl).

Inhibitor of Catechol-*O*-Methyl-Transferase (COMT)

COMT is an enzyme that degrades levodopa, and blocking it raises the levels of circulating levodopa. The primary drug from this class is entacapone (Comtan). Entacapone is only used concurrently with carbidopa/levodopa. When combined with carbidopa/levodopa in a single pill, it is sold as the brand name Stalevo.

Treatment Guidelines

These drugs have a place in the treatment of Parkinson's disease; however, advanced Parkinson's disease with dementia or DLB requires a simplified strategy. In this context, the benefit of medications can be offset by side effects, such as hallucinations or delusions. Visual hallucinations and, to a lesser extent, delusions (bizarre beliefs, paranoia, etc.) often occur spontaneously in these disorders. However, they can also be provoked by dopamine-replenishing drugs.

Below are basic clinical facts that should guide treatment selection.

1. Levodopa (carbidopa/levodopa) is by far the most efficacious of these dopamine-enhancing drugs.

2. Carbidopa/levodopa by itself is often well tolerated in DLB or PDD if used alone, but the risk of hallucinations increases substantially if another dopamine-enhancing drug is added to it.

3. The dopamine agonist drugs ropinirole (Requip), pramipexole (Mirapex), and rotigotine (Neupro) are less efficacious than levodopa. In clinical trials they were approximately three times as likely to provoke hallucinations.

4. Adding entacapone (Comtan) to carbidopa/levodopa (Stalevo) slightly increases the risk of hallucinations and markedly adds to the cost of treatment.

5. The MAO-B inhibitor drugs, rasagiline (Azilect) and selegiline, are much less effective at treating parkinsonism than either levodopa or the dopamine agonists.

The conclusion is that in DLB or PDD, carbidopa/levodopa by itself is the best medication strategy. Parenthetically, it also is the least expensive, by far. Carbidopa/levodopa has been off patent for many years, and the generic formulation is a relatively inexpensive medication. Dopamine agonists (pramipexole, ropinirole, rotigotine) are sometimes tried in the setting of DLB and PDD; however, the side effects, lesser efficacy, and expense outweigh the benefits.

Among the alternatives to carbidopa/levodopa, the dopamine agonists (pramipexole, ropinirole, and rotigotine) are the next most efficacious in treating parkinsonism. However, they have unique side effects:

1. Provocation of compulsive gambling, eating, spending, or sexual pursuits, often in people with no prior proclivities
2. Sleepiness
3. Leg swelling (edema), which is not worrisome but occasionally is severe

As mentioned earlier, they are also more likely than plain carbidopa/levodopa to provoke hallucinations or delusions. The dopamine agonist drugs are also much more expensive than carbidopa/levodopa.

DRUGS FOR PARKINSONISM TARGETING OTHER NEUROTRANSMITTERS

Some older drugs for parkinsonism work through brain neurotransmitters other than dopamine, and these deserve comment here.

Medications blocking the neurotransmitter acetylcholine were the primary drugs for treating Parkinson's disease before levodopa was identified. These drugs are called anticholinergics. They are a particularly bad choice in DLB and PDD because acetylcholine is a neurotransmitter in brain memory circuits. Blocking brain acetylcholine may impair memory and elicit hallucinations. This class of drugs has several other common side effects; they are best avoided in this setting. Two common drugs from this class are trihexyphenidyl (Artane) and benztropine (Cogentin).

Amantadine became available for treating parkinsonism around the time that levodopa was introduced, around 40 years ago, and it is still used today. As discussed in Chapter 8, it is primarily prescribed for reducing certain involuntary movements (dyskinesias). Otherwise, it is no more than mildly

beneficial for treating parkinsonism. It may promote hallucinations and is best reserved for those uncommon situations in
which dyskinesias cannot be controlled by other means. Even
then, it might not be advisable to use it in people highly prone
to hallucinations.

BOTTOM LINE: WHICH DRUG FOR PARKINSONISM IN DLB OR PDD?

The safest, cheapest, and most efficacious drug for replenish-
ing dopamine in this situation is carbidopa/levodopa. Various
names for this are used interchangeably. Sometimes it is simply termed "levodopa" or "l-dopa." The brand name Sinemet
is also used, even though it has been off patent for years and
the prescription is conventionally filled with the generic form.
This is the sole drug advocated in this book for treating parkinsonism. The next chapter addresses when and how to use it in
these disorders.

ONE LAST THING: DRUGS THAT BLOCK DOPAMINE

Whereas drugs that improve dopamine neurotransmission are
beneficial, drugs that block dopamine have the opposite effect
and can cause parkinsonism, even in normal people. Drugs that
block brain dopamine are from the two classes listed below and
should be avoided.

Medications for Nausea

Metoclopramide (Reglan) and prochlorperazine (Compazine)
are dopamine blockers used to treat nausea; they should
be avoided in the setting of DLB or PDD. Antinausea drugs
that are acceptable include trimethobenzamide (Tigan) and
ondansetron (Zofran). Outside the United States, domperidone

is frequently prescribed for nausea. It does not get into the brain, so that even though it blocks dopamine, it does not worsen parkinsonism.

Medications for Psychosis

The medications generally used to treat certain psychiatric thought disorders are called neuroleptics or antipsychotics (e.g., haloperidol, risperidone, and many others). Although these drugs effectively treat hallucinations and delusions, most of them block dopamine receptors, potentially causing parkinsonism. Two drugs from this class that do not provoke parkinsonism are quetiapine (Seroquel) and clozapine (Clozaril). As discussed in more detail in Chapter 10, quetiapine is an appropriate choice in DLB and PDD when hallucinations cannot be controlled through simpler strategies.

6

Beginning Carbidopa/Levodopa Treatment

Background, Starting Dosages, and Side Effects

In the previous chapter the symptoms and signs of parkinsonism were described, along with the rationale for selecting carbidopa/levodopa as the primary drug for treating parkinsonism. In most cases of DLB or PDD, carbidopa/levodopa should be the only drug used for dopamine replenishment. This strategy results in the greatest likelihood of substantial benefits and least risk of side effects. If parkinsonism is minimal and causing no disability, carbidopa/levodopa does not need to be started.

Certain non-motor parkinsonism symptoms in DLB and PDD may also respond to carbidopa/levodopa treatment, including anxiety, insomnia, and sometimes pain. Treatment of these non-motor symptoms will be discussed in Chapter 9.

This chapter outlines levodopa treatment guidelines for people whose parkinsonism is troublesome and untreated. The guidelines presented here are also relevant to those taking only low doses of carbidopa/levodopa.

If other drugs are being taken for parkinsonism it may be wise to begin tapering those off, one by one, before adding carbidopa/levodopa. This process is addressed in further detail in Chapter 7. Tapering off other drugs for parkinsonism should not be done without the clinician's input. Drugs to consider for slow elimination include ropinirole (Requip), pramipexole (Mirapex), rotigotine (Neupro patch), selegiline (Eldepryl), rasagiline (Azilect), benztropine (Cogentin), and trihexyphenidyl (Artane). Amantadine may also fall into this category, although there are circumstances where it may be indicated (for hard-to-treat dyskinesias). Entacapone, taken as either Comtan or Stalevo, is also addressed in the next chapter.

This chapter begins with a discussion of basic facts and principles relating to carbidopa/levodopa, before outlining specific treatment algorithms. The chapter ends with a discussion of possible side effects. Carbidopa/levodopa is usually well tolerated, as long as it is not combined with other parkinsonism drugs.

WHAT IS CARBIDOPA/LEVODOPA?

The active ingredient in this formulation is levodopa. Everyone has levodopa in their bodies, and small amounts are present in the diet. This natural substance is the precursor to dopamine. An enzyme, dopa decarboxylase, is present in the brain and body that converts levodopa to dopamine.

When ingested, levodopa enters the bloodstream via the stomach to the small intestine, then into the circulation. From the bloodstream it can be transported into the brain, where it is taken up by appropriate brain cells. There it can be stored and converted to dopamine by the enzyme dopa decarboxylase.

Dopamine itself cannot get into the brain, so it is not used to treat parkinsonism. Dopamine cannot cross from the bloodstream into the brain because of a barrier, appropriately called the blood–brain barrier. However, levodopa is easily picked up by a special transport system at the blood–brain barrier. This biological transporter specifically recognizes levodopa and related natural compounds, selecting them for passage into the brain.

Levodopa alone can be an effective treatment for parkinsonism, but without carbidopa it does not work as well. The problem is that levodopa is easily transformed to dopamine prematurely, outside the brain. The enzyme that converts levodopa to dopamine (dopa decarboxylase) is also present in the bloodstream and other organs; hence, circulating levodopa is easily converted to dopamine by that enzyme outside the brain. This premature conversion to dopamine results in two undesirable outcomes:

1. Prematurely formed dopamine cannot cross the blood–brain barrier and, hence, cannot restore brain dopamine levels.
2. Dopamine in the circulation penetrates one small region where the blood–brain barrier is patent: the nausea/vomiting center.

Restated, levodopa without carbidopa generates a lot of circulating dopamine (but much less brain dopamine). This gets trapped outside the brain and stimulates the nausea center, tending to induce vomiting.

When levodopa was first introduced decades ago, it was administered alone (without carbidopa). Nausea and vomiting were common, and large levodopa doses were necessary to overcome this premature conversion to dopamine. Scientists recognized the problem and designed a drug, carbidopa, which has two properties:

1. It blocks dopa decarboxylase.
2. It does not cross the blood–brain barrier.

Thus, carbidopa blocks dopa decarboxylase, but only outside the brain. With carbidopa, much smaller levodopa doses can be used. More importantly, nausea is avoided because less dopamine is being generated before passage across the blood–brain barrier. It is the dopamine in the bloodstream that stimulates the brain stem nausea center (which has no blood–brain barrier). Interestingly, the brand name applied to this new drug in the 1970s was Sinemet, derived from the Latin *sine*, meaning without, and *emesis*, meaning vomiting (i.e., without vomiting). Carbidopa/levodopa has been the standard treatment of Parkinson's disease for four decades and is also crucial for treating certain aspects of DLB. A drug nearly identical to carbidopa, benserazide, is similarly used in some countries outside the United States (benserazide/levodopa). What is written about carbidopa/levodopa in this book applies similarly to benserazide/levodopa.

FORMULATIONS OF CARBIDOPA/LEVODOPA

Carbidopa/levodopa pills come in three different forms:

1. Regular (often termed "immediate-release")
2. Sustained-release (SR), or controlled-release (CR)
3. Dispersible, which is a form that dissolves in the mouth and is swallowed with the saliva

In this book, we will use the first formulation, the regular carbidopa/levodopa; it is also termed immediate-release to distinguish it from the controlled-release drug.

Why Choose the Regular, Immediate-Release Form of Carbidopa/Levodopa?

Regular (immediate-release) carbidopa/levodopa is cheaper, easier to use, and more predictable; it results in less erratic responses than the CR formulation. In contrast to regular carbidopa/levodopa, the CR drug takes twice as long to work and has complex interactions with food; thus there are more complex rules governing how to use it. Sometimes people wrongly assume that if they use the sustained-release formulation of carbidopa/levodopa they would only need to take it once daily. However, that is not correct; the sustained-release properties only increase the levodopa effect by 60 to 90 minutes. Hence, we will focus on treating parkinsonism with regular (immediate-release) carbidopa/levodopa.

At the time of publication of this book, another extended-release carbidopa/levodopa formulation was being studied in clinical trials, initially designated by the investigational number IPX066. It is expected to be approved by the U.S. Food and Drug Administration by the end of 2013 and will probably be marketed under the brand name Rytary, This capsule contains combinations of immediate-release and sustained-release carbidopa/levodopa. The early experience suggests that it may indeed benefit those with more advanced problems and unsustained levodopa responses. However, dosing will be more complicated and it will undoubtedly be much more expensive; it will not be necessary for initial therapy. Since the experience with this carbidopa/levodopa formulation is preliminary, we will not address it further in this text.

Finally, there is a dispersible form of carbidopa/levodopa (Parcopa), which can be used interchangeably with the immediate-release form but is much more expensive. It quickly dissolves in the mouth and is swallowed with the saliva; it may get into the system slightly faster than the regular form, but not dramatically quicker. Given the greater expense, we will not promote this form either.

Dosages of Regular (Immediate-Release) and CR Carbidopa/Levodopa Are Not Interchangeable

Occasionally, dosing mistakes are made when someone tries to convert from regular carbidopa/levodopa to the CR (sustained-release) formulation or vice versa. They do NOT have a milligram (mg)-to-milligram correspondence. This is because the sustained-release (SR or CR) form only partially passes into the circulation and is released at a slower rate. To convert from regular carbidopa/levodopa to the CR drug, a 30 to 50% increase in the levodopa dosage is necessary (i.e., 200 mg of levodopa in the immediate-release form is approximately equivalent to 300 mg of the sustained-release formulation).

What if the patient is already on the CR form of carbidopa/levodopa? In general, if this person is doing well, then it is reasonable to not rock the boat. However, if it seems that levodopa adjustments will be necessary, it may be desirable to work with the clinician to switch to the immediate-release formulation. Again, when making such a switch, it is important to remember that 300 mg of levodopa in the sustained-release form equates to about 200 mg in regular carbidopa/levodopa. Converting this may take some trial-and-error adjustments.

Regular (Immediate-Release) Carbidopa/Levodopa Pill Sizes

The pill size is specified in two numbers: the first is the carbidopa amount in milligrams, and the second, levodopa. Thus, a 25/100 pill contains 25 mg of carbidopa and 100 mg of levodopa. The amount of carbidopa is important only if nausea is a problem. Otherwise it can be ignored; most people require only relatively small amounts of carbidopa to control nausea, and larger amounts (even very large amounts) of carbidopa cause no problems. The active ingredient that directly leads to brain dopamine replenishment is levodopa, which is the second number in the pill size. Thus, pill potency relates to this number.

There are three sizes of regular carbidopa/levodopa:

10/100
This is slightly cheaper than the more commonly used 25/100 size (see below); however, because there is less carbidopa, it is less likely to control nausea. If nausea is not present, this form may be used.

25/100

The larger amount of carbidopa in this formulation makes this a better choice because it controls nausea better. This is the formulation we will primarily recommend in this book.

25/250

This pill has two and a half times the amount of levodopa as the above two formulations. It is not used initially, since levodopa should be started with lesser amounts and small dosage increases are not possible. However, it may be used in place of two and a half tablets of the 25/100 (or 10/100) sizes, provided that the lesser amount of carbidopa does not result in nausea. Note that the 25/250 size can be broken in half and used for more gradual dosage escalation. Thus, one-half of a 25/250 tablet provides 125 mg of levodopa. Similarly, combining this half of a 25/250 tablet (125 mg levodopa) with one-half of a 25/100 pill (50 mg levodopa) yields 175 mg of levodopa. These pills are generally scored in the middle to make them easy to break in half.

What about Starting with Stalevo?

Stalevo is another form of carbidopa/levodopa and has a third drug added to it, entacapone; that is, Stalevo is the combination of carbidopa, levodopa, and entacapone. It is a little more complicated to use than plain carbidopa/levodopa and much more expensive. Note that entacapone is administered in only one amount, 200 mg; larger entacapone doses do not increase the potency. Thus, if entacapone is desired, it may be easier to provide a separate 200 mg entacapone pill and make dose adjustments with carbidopa/levodopa alone. People with DLB or PDD have potential for developing hallucinations, and adding adjunctive drugs to carbidopa/levodopa may promote such problems. Hence, we will not advocate using entacapone in this book, although there may be rare exceptions when this is beneficial and tolerated in individuals with DLB or PDD.

GUIDELINES FOR PEOPLE ON NO OTHER PARKINSONISM DRUGS

The next sections provide instructions for beginning carbidopa/ levodopa and are appropriate if the person is taking no other medications for parkinsonism. Other drugs for parkinsonism complicate treatment and require further advice, contained in Chapter 7. Thus, if the patient is taking rasagiline (Azilect), sele- giline (Eldepryl), pramipexole (Mirapex), ropinirole (Requip), Stalevo, trihexyphenidyl, benztropine, or amantadine, then the next chapter should also be read before starting carbidopa/ levodopa.

GENERAL PRINCIPLES: STARTING CARBIDOPA/LEVODOPA TREATMENT

Carbidopa/Levodopa Must be Taken on an Empty Stomach

Levodopa must cross the blood–brain barrier to get into the brain, where it is then converted to dopamine. It crosses the blood–brain barrier by being picked up by a special transporter mechanism that binds to amino acids, carrying them across this barrier. Levodopa is an amino acid; dopamine is not, so it will not be transported.

Meals come into play in the administration of carbidopa/ levodopa because of potential competition from dietary pro- teins (e.g., meat, fish, milk, cheese, beans, poultry). Proteins are made up of strings of amino acids. When proteins are digested, the constituent amino acids are liberated into the bloodstream. They then can compete with levodopa for binding sites on the transporter mechanism. This transporter molecule recognizes a whole class of amino acids and has only limited carrying capac- ity. Hence, if dietary amino acids fill up all the binding sites, levodopa cannot "get a seat."

Carbidopa/levodopa is not harmful to the stomach or intestine. Recall that the nausea is not due to irritation of the stomach lining, but rather to stimulation of the brainstem nausea center.

How Separate from Meals Must Carbidopa/Levodopa Doses be Taken?

Patients who are very sensitive to the meal effects of the drug have taught us that the carbidopa/levodopa doses should be taken

- At least an hour before a meal
- At least 2 hours after the end of a meal

If it is taken too close to a meal, some of the levodopa effect will be lost, and occasionally the whole effect is lost. Conventionally, carbidopa/levodopa is started with a three-times-daily scheme and administered about an hour (or more) before each of the three meals. If a meal is skipped, obviously, it may be taken at any time.

Carbidopa/levodopa Dosage Escalation

Throughout this book, the 25/100 size of the regular (immediate-release) formulation will be advised and discussed. It should be taken on an empty stomach for the full effect, as stipulated above. By convention, this medication is taken three times daily; hence dosing an hour before each of three meals is a simple way to remember this. If a meal is skipped, it may be taken at any time.

The starting dose is either one-half or a full 25/100 tablet, taken three times daily. In my clinic, I have people start with a full tablet, three times daily. However, most people will not appreciate a substantial benefit on that dosage; higher doses are usually necessary for the full benefit.

It takes about a week or slightly longer for the benefit from a given dosage to slowly develop and plateau. Typically, I have people raise the dosage at weekly intervals, guided by their response. An easy way to escalate the dosage is by adding a half-tablet to all three doses every week. Thus, for the second week, one and a half tablets are taken three times daily; the third week, two tablets three times daily, and so on.

There is potential for further benefit from up to three tablets each dose; however, most people will have developed the full effect by the time they get up to two and a half tablets each dose. With this in mind, the dosing scheme that I recommend starts with one tablet three times daily and ends with a dosage of two and a half tablets three times daily. If it appears that further benefit is necessary, I do allow people to go to three tablets each dose, but only if there are no side effects. Restated, there is potential for incremental benefit with up to three tablets each dose; higher doses, such as four or five tablets each dose, provide no further improvement (provided using the 25/100 immediate-release formulation, taken on an empty stomach). Side effects are discussed at the end of this chapter.

On any given dosage, it takes a week or a little longer for the full effect to slowly accumulate, so it is important to not give up on a dosage until it has been taken it for at least that long (if tolerated).

What Symptoms Should Be Targeted for Improvement?

The symptoms of parkinsonism (outlined in Chapter 4) are the primary reason for dopamine replenishment therapy with carbidopa/levodopa. However, as discussed in Chapter 9, anxiety and insomnia may also respond to this treatment. Furthermore, pain from any source may be more tolerable with adequate levodopa therapy. The overall goal is to keep people as active and ambulatory as possible. For those with less advanced parkinsonism, this would include levodopa dosages sufficient to allow regular exercise. However, even those with quite advanced disease with immobility may improve their ability to walk short distances or transfer better from bed to chair. Do not underestimate the potential benefit of carbidopa/levodopa to improve mobility.

SPECIFIC INSTRUCTIONS FOR INITIATING CARBIDOPA/LEVODOPA TREATMENT

If the treating physician agrees, dosage starts by taking one regular 25/100 carbidopa/levodopa tablet at least 1 hour before each of three meals; then follow the dose escalation scheme shown in Box 6.1. If side effects develop, the dosage does not need to be raised higher until those have been addressed. Most people will not experience troublesome side effects as they follow this dose escalation scheme.

As shown in Box 6.1, the dosage should go no higher than three tablets each dose. While higher doses are not dangerous, no further benefit will be achieved; the point of diminished returns is reached at that dose level. The primary principle is to settle on the dosage that works best. One may go all the way through the scheme and then return to a lower dosage if that was as effective as a higher dosage. Most people with Parkinson's disease going through this schedule will find that two or two and a half tablets each dose works best.

In the future, more doses may be necessary, which is discussed in detail in Chapter 8. However, for the first years of DLB or PD, the three doses are appropriate. When the Lewy disorder is long-standing (e.g., present beyond 5 to 8 years), most patients will need more frequent doses to avoid a decline in response between doses (see Chapter 8). When this adjustment seems appropriate, the milligram amount per dose will remain the same but will be taken at shorter intervals, with more doses per day.

Box 6.1 Starting Carbidopa/Levodopa 25/100 Regular (Immediate-Release) Pills

---

Take three doses daily. Take them on an empty stomach, at least an hour before meals. If you skip a meal, then take the dose at any time.

Week 1: One tablet 3 times daily
Week 2: One and a half tablets 3 times daily
Week 3: Two tablets 3 times daily
Week 4: Two and a half tablets 3 times daily*
Final instructions: Settle on the most effective dosage. If several doses are equally beneficial, settle on the lowest of those equipotent dosages.

*If there are no side effects and there is insufficient benefit, you may go up to three tablets 3 times daily.

What to Do If There Is No Benefit

In patients with Lewy disorders and parkinsonism, benefit from carbidopa/levodopa is expected. Unfortunately, those who do not benefit despite adequate dosage will not likely improve with one of the other parkinsonism drugs.

If there is no benefit on the highest dosage shown in Box 6.1 (2½ to 3 tablets 3 times daily) taken for at least 2 weeks, it is important to check that everything has been done correctly. Verify that the immediate-release (regular) formulation of carbidopa/levodopa was employed. Nearly all the generic formulations of this are yellow pills; if they are not yellow, check with the pharmacist. Also, confirm that this has been taken on an empty stomach, at least a full hour before meals (and at least 2 hours after the end of meals).

If correct dosing was used but was ineffective, the carbidopa/levodopa may be rapidly tapered off by reversing the scheme shown in Box 6.1. The dosage may be reduced every 2 days or so, down to zero; that is, taper off the drug over about 7 to 10 days. Unfortunately, there are no other useful alternative drugs for parkinsonism.

EARLY SIDE EFFECTS FROM CARBIDOPA/LEVODOPA AND WHAT TO DO ABOUT THEM

Generally, few people experience significant side effects when carbidopa/levodopa is started. However, nausea and low blood pressure (BP) deserve comment, since these effects may be limiting and usually can be controlled. While hallucinations may be provoked, this is highly unlikely if other drugs for parkinsonism are not being used.

Nausea

As mentioned earlier, nausea from carbidopa/levodopa does not relate to irritation of the stomach lining but rather is mediated at the brain level. Hence there is no potential for ulcers. Mild nausea typically abates after days to weeks with continued carbidopa/levodopa dosing and is not a cause for concern. Abdominal pain is not an expected carbidopa/levodopa side effect. If the symptom is abdominal pain rather than nausea, then other causes should be considered.

Nausea from carbidopa/levodopa is dose related; higher doses, such as three tablets, are more likely to cause this. If the nausea is only present on the highest doses, a lesser dose may resolve this. However, if nausea is an early and troublesome problem, then other strategies, as outlined below, can be used.

Although carbidopa/levodopa should be taken on an empty stomach, it may be taken with non-protein foods; having food in the stomach may reduce nausea. It may be taken with soda crackers, dry bread, or part of a banana.

If the nausea is present and problematic on the starting dosage of carbidopa/levodopa shown in Box 6.1, then this dosing scheme needs to be modified. In that case, one should start with one-fourth or one-half of a carbidopa/levodopa tablet three times daily and increase weekly by adding one-fourth tablet to all three doses. Continue to add this one-quarter tablet to all 3 doses every week, as tolerated, but this will require many weeks to get the dosage high enough to capture benefit.

Carbidopa prevents nausea, but for some people the amount of carbidopa in a 25/100 pill of carbidopa/levodopa is not enough. An additional simple strategy for reducing levodopa nausea is to prescribe additional carbidopa. It is available by prescription as plain carbidopa without levodopa (Lodosyn). It comes in one tablet size, 25 mg. For those with substantial nausea, supplementary carbidopa can be combined with the lower/slower carbidopa/levodopa dosing scheme outlined in the preceding paragraph (starting with very low carbidopa/levodopa doses and increasing much more slowly). One to two Lodosyn (carbidopa) tablets should be taken with or before each dose of carbidopa/levodopa. There appears to be no adverse consequences of taking extra carbidopa, except for the expense.

The most commonly prescribed medications for nausea, metoclopramide (Reglan) and prochlorperazine (Compazine), cannot be used. They block brain dopamine. They will likely worsen parkinsonism and prevent levodopa from working.

The other available antinausea drugs, trimethobenzamide (Tigan) and ondansetron (Zofran), are compatible with Lewy disorders and may be tried; however, they are not highly effective in this setting. Outside the United States, domperidone is typically used for nausea among those with parkinsonism. It blocks dopamine but cannot get into the brain, so it is compatible with parkinsonian conditions.

Orthostatic Hypotension

Orthostatic hypotension implies a drop in the blood pressure (BP) in the standing position. Normally, one's BP is essentially the same whether sitting, lying, or standing. In these Lewy disorders, there is a variable tendency for this regulation to be lost or reduced, because these Lewy conditions also affect the autonomic nervous system (dysautonomia), as discussed in Chapter 4. In people with orthostatic hypotension, BP may be normal while sitting, but drop so low when they stand that they feel faint or actually faint. This tendency can be substantially exacerbated by carbidopa/levodopa. Detection of orthostatic hypotension is a key factor, since it cannot be treated if it is not recognized. When orthostatic hypotension surfaces it can be very troublesome, but it is treatable. An entire chapter is devoted to treating this problem: Chapter 13.

Most people with Lewy disorders will not have trouble with orthostatic hypotension, even with aggressive levodopa treatment. Nonetheless, proper vigilance regarding this potential problem is appropriate. Before starting carbidopa/levodopa, the standing and sitting BP should be checked. If the standing BP is already low, then caution is warranted.

At this juncture, background on BP seems appropriate; a more detailed discussion is found in Chapter 13. BP readings, such as 120/80, come in two numbers, with the first value called the systolic BP and the second, the diastolic BP. Typically, they run fairly parallel to each other, so to keep things simple in this text we will focus on the first number (systolic) and provide guidelines based on that.

A normal blood pressure is around 120/80, although normal (nonhypertensive) adults may have systolic values between 100 and 140. People tolerate systolic BP down to about 90. Anything much below that may be associated with faintness. If the systolic BP drops substantially below 70, faints or near faints tend to occur.

As a rule of thumb, the standing systolic BP should consistently be maintained above 90 to avoid faintness. However, since carbidopa/levodopa may lower the standing BP, ideally it should be a little higher than 90 before starting carbidopa/levodopa. Hence, before starting carbidopa/levodopa, standing BP should be checked. If this is less than 100 before carbidopa/levodopa is initiated, it may be wise to defer this medication and address the low BP first.

If the systolic BP is around 100 or less, the medication list should be reviewed with the doctor. There are many drugs that lower BP, and these are discussed in Chapter 13.

Systolic BP values between 100 and 120 before carbidopa/levodopa administration are not problematic, but they may still signal the potential for hypotension (low BP) with carbidopa/levodopa therapy. Thus, if the standing systolic BP is less than 120 before beginning carbidopa/levodopa, it should be checked regularly once this drug is initiated. When carbidopa/levodopa lowers the BP, it does this for a few hours after every dose; the BP then returns to baseline 2 to 4 hours later. Hence, the timing of these BP checks is important. If it is done many hours after a dose is taken, the low BP will resolve and go undetected. Note that the drop in BP relates to the amount of levodopa in each dose; higher doses will tend to lower it more. Meals tend to lower BP and exacerbate this problem (termed postprandial hypotension). Finally, a night's sleep tends to lower BP, and this tendency will persist for several hours after rising. With all of these factors in mind, the standing BP should be checked in the morning after breakfast. This will capture the lowest reading of the day because it comes on the heels of a night's sleep, a meal, and the carbidopa/levodopa dose taken an hour before the morning meal.

If readings for several days have been satisfactory, measurement may be discontinued. However, if there is a susceptibility to orthostatic hypotension (low standing BP), continue to check the BP:

1. for several days after each increase in the carbidopa/levodopa dose, and
2. whenever there is a feeling of lightheadedness.

When recording the BP, the position—sitting, lying, or standing—should also be documented. The doctor will use this information to guide treatment. Remember that it is the standing BP that tends to drop with carbidopa/levodopa, so that should be documented in these readings.

What should one do in the immediate term if the BP is very low and faintness is experienced? The answer is simple: the person should sit or lie down and wait for the levodopa effect on BP to pass; this will take 2 to 4 hours. By definition, the low BPs of orthostatic hypotension normalize when the person is lying down and usually with sitting.

The primary symptom of low BP is lightheadedness. Vertigo, which is a spinning sensation, is not a symptom of low BP. Vertigo provoked by turning or bending over is common in older adults. If the cause is uncertain, check the BP in the position in which dizziness is present; if the BP is above 90 systolic when the person is experiencing this dizziness, then the dizziness is not due to low BP.

Hallucinations

Unfortunately, visual hallucinations are common in DLB and PDD. What is meant by this is seeing things that are not there, such as illusory people in the house or yard. In Lewy disorders, these visual hallucinations are primarily due to the disease itself; however, certain drugs can exacerbate this problem.

The reason for selecting carbidopa/levodopa over other medications for parkinsonism is that it is the least likely agent to cause hallucinations. For example, clinical trials have

documented that the dopamine agonists (pramipexole or ropinirole) are approximately three times more likely to provoke
hallucinations than carbidopa/levodopa. Whereas carbidopa/
levodopa alone infrequently causes hallucinations, the addition
of another parkinsonism drug substantially increases that risk.
Thus it is advised that carbidopa/levodopa be used by itself.

If hallucinations do develop while initiating carbidopa/
levodopa, it may be appropriate to reduce or taper off the
carbidopa/levodopa to see if the hallucinations are part of the
disease or truly caused by the medication; however, the benefit
of carbidopa/levodopa will obviously be lost. This is another
situation where it is wise to review the medication list with the
clinician to make sure that no other drugs are contributing
to the occurrence of hallucinations. Sleep deprivation (due to
insomnia or untreated sleep apnea) may increase the tendency
toward hallucinations. Similarly, untreated illnesses as simple as
a urinary infection may also increase this tendency. If hallucinations need further treatment, see Chapter 10, which focuses
on this problem.

OUTSIDE THE UNITED STATES:
BENSERAZIDE INSTEAD OF CARBIDOPA

This book focuses on carbidopa/levodopa treatment for parkinsonism. Outside the United States, levodopa may be formulated
with a different dopa decarboxylase inhibitor, benserazide, in
place of carbidopa. Benserazide performs identically to carbidopa and is prescribed in the same milligram amount and
with the same ratio as in the 25/100 formulation of carbidopa/
levodopa (i.e., 25 mg of benserazide or carbidopa added to
100 mg of levodopa). However, the two most common brands
of benserazide and levodopa, Prolopa and Madopar, list the
milligram amounts differently from carbidopa/levodopa and
also from one another. This can be confusing and deserves
discussion.

Prolopa is available in Canada as well as in several other countries. Prolopa capsules list the milligrams of levodopa first, then benserazide. For example, the 100-25 size indicates 100 mg of levodopa and 25 mg of benserazide (equivalent to the 25/100 formulation of carbidopa/levodopa).

The Madopar brand of benserazide/levodopa is available in many countries outside of the United States and Canada, and the ingredients are listed differently from both carbidopa/levodopa and Prolopa. Madopar pill and capsule sizes are given as a single number, adding the milligram amounts of the two ingredients, benserazide and levodopa. The Madopar pill or capsule containing 100 mg of levodopa and 25 mg of benserazide is listed as "125 mg." Madopar 125 is equivalent to the 25/100 formulation of carbidopa/levodopa. Other formulations include Madopar 62.5 (50 mg of levodopa and 12.5 mg of benserazide) and Madopar 250 (200 mg of levodopa and 50 mg benserazide).

The guidelines in this book are also appropriate for people in countries where only levodopa with benserazide is available. However, one needs to understand how the ingredients are listed. Levodopa/benserazide will not be referred to further in this book, since carbidopa/levodopa is interchangeable with the benserazide-levodopa formulations. One simply needs to understand the different numbering systems for these two products.

7

Parkinsonism Treatment for Those Already on Medications

The previous chapter provided instructions for starting and adjusting carbidopa/levodopa, but specifically pertained to those individuals on no other drugs for parkinsonism or those on only a low carbidopa/levodopa dosage. In this chapter, we focus on people who are taking other drugs for parkinsonism either with or without carbidopa/levodopa.

As mentioned earlier, people with DLB or PDD are prone to hallucinations and delusions, which can be exacerbated by drugs for parkinsonism. Carbidopa/levodopa is the least likely to worsen or provoke these problems; however, this is true only if it is used alone (i.e., without other parkinsonism drugs). Carbidopa/levodopa is also the most efficacious drug for parkinsonism. Thus it is reasonable to take the approach that carbidopa/levodopa should be the sole treatment for parkinsonism in DLB or PDD.

Whereas using carbidopa/levodopa by itself is often tolerated, adding it to other parkinsonian medications may provoke problems, especially hallucinations or delusions. Hence, before starting carbidopa/levodopa, it is wise to scrutinize the medication list and eliminate other parkinsonism drugs, one by one.

There are two general rules of thumb regarding these medications:

1. It is not necessary to change drugs if things are going well and are expected to continue.
2. Change only one medication at a time (but if there are severe drug side effects, the physician may take more aggressive action).

Some drugs are worse offenders than others and will be prioritized with that in mind. Note that a variety of schemes may be employed to taper off a drug. The drug-elimination schedules provided below are somewhat arbitrary and other similar schedules may work as well. The most important factor is the total time to reduce the dosage down to zero. The longer a person has been on a medication and the higher the dosage, the more prolonged the taper. The clinician needs to work closely with the patient as this is being done. Parkinsonism may transiently worsen when these drugs are eliminated; however, this typically can subsequently be reversed with carbidopa/levodopa adjustments.

DRUGS TO ELIMINATE FIRST: ANTICHOLINERGICS

Trihexyphenidyl (Artane), Benztropine (Cogentin)

These anticholinergic drugs tend to impair memory and contribute to hallucinations and delusions; they are never a good choice in DLB or PDD. They also slow the gastrointestinal tract, aggravating constipation. If they have been started within the past 6 weeks, they can be tapered off over about a week. If started in the past year or two, they may be tapered off over 2 to 3 weeks. However, if these have been taken for years, then a slower taper should be considered. Allow an interval (perhaps a week) before starting or increasing carbidopa/levodopa after these have been stopped.

DRUGS TO ELIMINATE NEXT: DOPAMINE AGONISTS

Pramipexole (Mirapex), Ropinirole (Requip), Rotigotine (Neupro Patch)

The dopamine agonist drugs are more complicated to use than carbidopa/levodopa and less efficacious; they are especially prone to side effects in the context of DLB or PDD. In general, more rapid tapering is favored if important side effects surface, such as hallucinations, delusions, or serious behavioral compulsions (e.g., gambling, shopping, sexual behaviors). However, some people experience withdrawal (e.g., severe anxiety, pain, or depression), which may require much slower tapering.

General schemes for discontinuation are outlined below, but these are general guidelines and may require either more rapid or slower tapering, depending on the circumstances. Talk with the clinician to be sure it is done correctly. Note that pramipexole and ropinirole are formulated in both a regular-release pill and an extended-release (once-daily) form. The extended-release formulations are easier to taper and are discussed separately, below.

Pramipexole (Mirapex), regular-release (not extended-release). This can be rapidly tapered if the dosage is low, such as 0.25 mg three times daily or less. To taper off that dosage, reduce all doses by half for 5 days, then eliminate one of the three doses every other day until completely off the drug. For pramipexole dosages of 0.375 to 0.5 three times daily, extend the taper to 2 to 3 weeks. Dosages much higher than that require 3 to 4 weeks of tapering. Occasional patients may develop withdrawal symptoms if starting from high doses, and may require an even slower taper. Carbidopa/levodopa may be started about a week after the pramipexole is stopped. An interval between pramipexole (or other drug) discontinuation and carbidopa/levodopa initiation is advisable so that withdrawal symptoms are not inappropriately attributed to carbidopa/levodopa.

Ropinirole (Requip), regular-release (not extended-release). This dopamine agonist is tapered similarly to pramipexole, although the milligram (mg) amounts are not equivalent between these two drugs. A low ropinirole dosage of 1 mg three times daily or less can be tapered quickly over about 7 to 10 days. Ropinirole pills cannot be cut in half so the clinician will need to prescribe lower-dose pill sizes. A dosage of up to 2 mg three times daily should be tapered off over approximately 2 to 3 weeks, and doses of 3 mg to 5 mg taken three times daily can be tapered off over a month or so.

Pramipexole, extended-release (Mirapex ER). Tapering off this sustained-release formulation will require multiple dose sizes of pills from the clinician. Pills should not be broken in half because this changes the release rate. The duration for tapering will approximate what was cited earlier for the regular formulations of pramipexole; the milligrams *per day* are essentially the same for the regular and the extended-release formulations of this drug. The extended-release sizes are 4.5 mg, 3.75 mg, 3 mg, 2.25 mg, 1.5 mg, 0.75 mg, and 0.375 mg, each taken once daily. A simple strategy is to reduce weekly by going to the next lower pill size. When a patient is on 0.375 mg once daily for a week, the drug can be stopped.

Ropinirole, extended-release (Requip XL). As with extended-release pramipexole, the clinician will need to provide prescriptions for smaller pill sizes to allow tapering (do not halve the pills). It comes in five sizes: 12 mg, 8 mg, 6 mg, 4 mg, and 2 mg. The simplest strategy is to reduce the dosage by 2 mg each week until off the drug.

Rotigotine patch (Neupro). If a single 1 mg or 2 mg patch is being used, it may be stopped without further taper. Higher daily dosages can be tapered by eliminating 2 mg each week. The clinician may need to provide prescriptions for different patch sizes to allow tapering. It comes in 1 mg, 2 mg, 3 mg, 4 mg, 6 mg, and 8 mg patch sizes. Note that a milligram of rotigotine is approximately similar in potency to a milligram of ropinirole. In other words, 6 mg of rotigotine and 6 mg of ropinirole have similar effects.

Pramipexole and ropinirole are also used in the evening and bedtime to treat restless legs syndrome. Much lower dosages are used for that purpose, carrying a lesser risk of hallucinations. This treatment may be acceptable, provided hallucinations and delusions remain absent.

OTHER DRUGS THAT MAY PROVOKE HALLUCINATIONS, ESPECIALLY WHEN ADDED TO CARBIDOPA/LEVODOPA

Rasagiline (Azilect), Selegiline

These MAO-B inhibitors are sometimes advocated because of the conviction that they slow disease progression. However, there is no compelling evidence for this, and the FDA has declined approval for that purpose in the context of Parkinson's disease. They are only mildly helpful in treating parkinsonism. When combined with carbidopa/levodopa, they may provoke hallucinations or delusions. It makes sense to eliminate these sooner rather than later in the setting of DLB or PDD.

Rasagiline (Azilect) and selegiline can be stopped abruptly. They have a very long duration of action in the brain, with a half-life of 40 days. Hence, no tapering is necessary. After discontinuation, carbidopa/levodopa can be started or increased a week later. If hallucinations subsequently occur, this could be due to the residual effect of rasagiline or selegiline because of their long half-lives. In that case, the carbidopa/levodopa should be reduced or stopped and then retried perhaps 2 to 3 months later.

AMANTADINE

Amantadine is an older drug that previously was used to treat very mild cases of Parkinson's disease. However, it is not very efficacious for parkinsonism and can occasionally provoke hallucinations. The current primary use for amantadine is to reduce levodopa-related dyskinesias, the involuntary chaotic body movements due to an excessive levodopa effect. These dance-like movements need to be distinguished from tremor or dystonia and are described in Chapter 8. The primary strategy for eliminating dyskinesias is to reduce the individual doses of carbidopa/levodopa, whereas amantadine is used when carbidopa/levodopa dose reduction results in increased parkinsonism. That is a very uncommon problem among people with DLB or PDD.

To summarize: if dyskinesias (involuntary dance-like movements) are not a problem, taper off amantadine. Amantadine comes in one size, 100-mg tablets. A simple tapering strategy is to eliminate one of these tablets each week until completely discontinued. However, if dyskinesias are problematic and amantadine seems necessary, it may be continued if no hallucinations or delusions are present. See Chapter 8 for a detailed discussion of dyskinesia treatment.

COMT INHIBITOR: UNNECESSARY AND EXPENSIVE

Entacapone (Comtan)

Catechol-*O*-methyltransferase (COMT) is an enzyme that degrades levodopa; it is blocked by entacapone. Entacapone is only used in conjunction with carbidopa/levodopa and does not affect parkinsonism if used alone. It enables levodopa to remain in the bloodstream 30 to 60 minutes longer and produces a slightly more potent response. It is unnecessary for most people with DLB or PDD and may complicate treatment.

Entacapone (Comtan) comes in one size, 200 mg, and is taken with each dose of carbidopa/levodopa. There is no purpose in taking more or less than 200 mg for each dose. The enhancement of levodopa lasts for about 4 hours after each dose. Entacapone is also formulated in the same pill with carbidopa/levodopa, prescribed as brand name Stalevo.

There are several reasons for eliminating entacapone and using only carbidopa/levodopa: (1) entacapone is expensive; (2) it is slightly more complicated to use; (3) the benefits are not substantially different from simply taking a higher dosage of carbidopa/levodopa, except for lasting 30 to 60 minutes longer; (4) it may have a slight tendency to provoke hallucinations but probably less than the other drugs listed above.

If taking entacapone as a separate pill, it may be stopped abruptly. The levodopa effect may slightly diminish but if problematic can usually be restored by raising the carbidopa/levodopa by a half-tablet (25/100) each dose.

Stalevo is a combination pill that includes entacapone (200 mg) plus carbidopa/levodopa. If used, it can be switched to plain carbidopa/levodopa, using the same amount of levodopa. Note that Stalevo-100 is entacapone plus 25/100 carbidopa/levodopa; Stalevo-200 is entacapone plus the equivalent of two 25/100 carbidopa/levodopa tablets, and so on. Every Stalevo tablet contains 200 mg of entacapone, regardless of the amount of carbidopa or levodopa. Thus, if a patient is taking Stalevo-200 each dose, the person may switch to two of the 25/100 pills of regular (immediate-release) carbidopa/levodopa. If each dose is Stalevo-100, the person can switch to one tablet of immediate-release carbidopa/levodopa (25/100).

Tolcapone is another COMT inhibitor that is rarely prescribed because it has potential to cause serious liver damage. It requires close monitoring of liver function tests, if prescribed. This drug will not be discussed further in this text.

WHAT NEXT?

Once off these other drugs it should then be possible to initiate or adjust the carbidopa/levodopa dosage according to the guidelines in Chapter 6. Usually, this can be done without provoking hallucinations or delusions, once the other parkinsonism drugs have been discontinued. However, if hallucinations or delusions develop despite medication simplification, refer to Chapter 10 for strategies directed at treating these conditions.

8

Unstable Responses and Dyskinesias

Later Motor Problems

Chapter 6 outlined the symptoms that should benefit from carbidopa/levodopa treatment and how to initiate it. Once the optimum dosing scheme has been established there usually is not much medication adjustment required for the initial few years. However, this situation changes with longer durations of DLB or Parkinson's disease.

During the first several years of DLB or Parkinson's disease, treatment with carbidopa/levodopa is straightforward—the responses are stable and unchanging over the course of the day. Thus, the exact time a person takes the doses is not important as long as they are administered on an empty stomach (at least 1 hour before and 2 hours after meals). If the dosage is changed, it takes about a week for the response to fully develop. This pattern of a stable levodopa response that slowly accumulates over a week is termed the long-duration response.

LONG-DURATION RESPONSE

For this response to fully develop and capture the maximum benefit, about six to eight tablets of the regular (immediate-release) carbidopa/levodopa 25/100 tablets per day are necessary. While this has not been well studied in clinical trials, experience in the clinic suggests that this is approximately correct.

After a few years of having DLB or Parkinson's disease, the person's response to levodopa tends to change. The long-duration effect persists, but part of the benefit becomes time-locked to each dose. This response does not reflect how long the person has been taking carbidopa/levodopa but how long he or she has had DLB or Parkinson's disease. As these conditions progress, the capacity to maintain a stable, around-the-clock effect from levodopa diminishes, as if the effect could no longer be stored-up. This is not simply a brain levodopa storage problem, but it behaves that way. People with this time-locked benefit from levodopa will note that their gait, stiffness, tremor, and slowness will improve an hour or so after taking a carbidopa/levodopa dose. In other words, it takes about an hour (sometimes less) for the regular carbidopa/levodopa to "kick in." Initially, this benefit may last 4 to 5 hours, but after many years it may diminish to 2 hours or less. This effect that is time-locked to each dose of carbidopa/levodopa is termed the short-duration response.

SHORT-DURATION RESPONSE

Sometimes this response surfaces early, after only a year or two, but usually it is not very apparent until 5 to 8 years have elapsed. This time frame reflects the natural progression of these Lewy disorders.

This change in response pattern is often overlooked. Patients may report to their doctor that they can no longer walk well, or that the medicine (carbidopa/levodopa) no longer works, overlooking the fact that they actually experience control of symptoms during portions of the day. Wearing-off of the levodopa effect is the problem.

Savvy clinicians will ask such patients whether this loss of levodopa benefit has a pattern: are the problems occurring hours after their last dose, or close to the time for the next dose? It is crucial to establish that pattern, as this becomes the basis for levodopa dosage adjustments. Sometimes the pattern is most obvious following the first carbidopa/levodopa dose in the morning. Although occasional people are best after a night's sleep, most with this short-duration pattern experience a levodopa "off" state in the morning because they took no carbidopa/levodopa overnight. Thus, walking and movement are more difficult until the first dose of carbidopa/levodopa is taken and has a chance to work (usually taking about an hour). Observation at this time may provide the important clues: once carbidopa/levodopa kicks in, how long does the effect last? Typically, the durations of levodopa responses are quite reproducible; after assessment of a few such cycles, a fairly reliable estimate of the usual response-duration is possible. Did it last 4 hours, 3 hours?

Why is this important? It is because the duration of the levodopa response determines the appropriate dosing interval. Higher levodopa doses do not last substantially longer, even though intuition might suggest that. Thus, once the optimum amount of carbidopa/levodopa per dose is established (i.e., 2 tablets, 2½ tablets, etc.), this becomes the dose used indefinitely. It is the dosing interval that should change to treat the wearing-off of the levodopa effect.

Parkinsonism Is Not Controlled: More Levodopa per Dose or More Doses?

If parkinsonian symptoms (outlined in Chapter 6) are not adequately controlled, there are two treatable scenarios:

1. *Parkinsonism is poorly controlled all day long.* This suggests that the individual doses may be too low. In this circumstance more levodopa per dose is appropriate.
2. *Parkinsonism comes and goes, sometimes controlled, other times not.* This pattern suggests that the dosage is adequate to produce a good response (termed the "on"

response). However, the pattern may be that of wearing off, where the effect from a given dose does not last until the next dose.

The question is whether to take more per dose or to take the same dose more often. This needs to be addressed in more detail, since it is a crucial distinction.

Parkinsonism Is Poorly Controlled All Day Long, Despite Carbidopa/Levodopa

With this problem, it is unclear whether a short-duration response is potentially present, since control of parkinsonism is inadequate throughout the waking day. The appropriate strategy here is to gradually increase all the individual doses. It is not necessary to take more than three doses per day in this situation, each at least an hour before meals (or four doses, with the last at bedtime). Recall from Chapter 6 that there is potentially an incremental benefit with up to three tablets of the 25/100 (regular, immediate-release) formulation for each dose. As previously outlined, one can raise the dosage by a half-tablet (25/100) for all three doses each week, going from one tablet to one and a half tablets each dose, then two, etc., up to three tablets each dose. Most people with DLB or PDD capture the full effect by the time they have reached two and a half tablets each dose, but it is reasonable to go up to three tablets, if necessary. If the individual doses are less than two and a half to three tablets then they should be raised weekly and the outcome observed. Note that the maximum dose is specified as three tablets, not because higher doses are toxic, but rather because that dose captures all the potential benefit; higher individual doses do not add benefit.

If there is still insufficient control of parkinsonism, check the basics:

- Is the carbidopa/levodopa pill the regular, immediate-release formulation (pills are yellow except for one brand that is blue)? If there is any doubt, double-check this with the pharmacist.

- Are the doses taken on an empty stomach, at least an hour before meals and at least 2 hours after the end of meals?

If the dosage is taken correctly and there is still poor control of parkinsonism, there are unfortunately no other good medication options and the patient is left with this outcome. If, on the other hand, the doses have been raised and the result is parkinsonism control that comes and goes, read on.

Parkinsonism Comes and Goes: Sometimes Controlled, Other Times Not

Varying control of parkinsonism suggests wearing off of the levodopa effect. The patient or caregiver needs to pay attention to the response once a carbidopa/levodopa dose has a chance to kick in. Typically, the kick-in is an hour or so after a carbidopa/levodopa dose. If at that time symptoms are controlled, then this last dose of carbidopa/levodopa was adequate. This is termed the "on" response. If the on response is not as good as expected, there is the option of raising the dosage up to two and a half tablets per dose (occasionally, three tablets will prove optimal).

If the on response is satisfactory but does not last until the next dose, this implies that the interval between doses is too long. In that case, the dosing interval should be reduced to match the response duration. More doses per day may then be necessary.

Should There be Concern about the Number of Tablets per Day?

No. As long as the dosage is adjusted according to individual needs, the number of doses or tablets taken daily is not a concern. Thus, if there is a good response to two tablets of carbidopa/levodopa that lasts 4 hours, the patient should take two tablets every 4 hours. There is no maximum number of tablets per day; the only stipulation is a maximum of three tablets per dose.

Carbidopa/Levodopa at Bedtime or During the Night?

With a short-duration response, the patient will likely need coverage extending to and through the night in order to sleep well. Typically, this would include a dose at bedtime to get to sleep and perhaps a dose during the night if one awakens. The same amount of carbidopa/levodopa should be used for these nighttime doses. A common mistake is to assume that because you are asleep you can get by with less. That does not work. This is addressed in further detail in Chapter 9.

Side Effects from Carbidopa/Levodopa: All Have the Short-Duration Pattern

Fortunately, carbidopa/levodopa is usually tolerated without many side effects, provided it is not combined with other parkinsonism drugs. When side effects do occur, they have a short-duration pattern, as described above for levodopa benefits. In other words, the side effects are time-locked to each dose, lasting a few hours and then abating. A carbidopa/levodopa dose taken yesterday is not the cause of problems today. This knowledge is crucial to distinguishing levodopa-related side effects from effects due to other causes. If adverse symptoms persist for many hours (e.g., more than 6 hours) after the last carbidopa/levodopa dose, then other causes should be considered.

Side effects that may well be due to carbidopa/levodopa were discussed in Chapter 6 and include the following:

• Nausea
• Orthostatic hypotension (low blood pressure when standing or walking)
• Hallucinations
• Dyskinesias (involuntary movements, discussed next in this chapter)

Recognition that carbidopa/levodopa side effects have a short-duration pattern enables strategies for reducing their impact by changing the dosing times. For example, if one is susceptible to levodopa-induced nausea and there is concern that this may sabotage an evening at a restaurant, the next carbidopa/levodopa dose can be deferred until 2 hours after dinner. Any nausea from the prior lunchtime dose should have worn off by dinnertime. Or, if levodopa-induced orthostatic hypotension (low blood pressure when standing) threatens grocery shopping, similarly, a dose can be delayed until after standing in the checkout line. As discussed in Chapter 6 and later in this book, there are other more definitive measures for dealing with levodopa side effects, including dyskinesias, which are addressed next.

DYSKINESIAS

Dyskinesias are more prevalent among young people with Parkinson's disease. They are usually not very troublesome among most people with DLB or PDD. Moreover, if they do occur, they are treatable.

Dyskinesias are involuntary movements provoked by a dose of carbidopa/levodopa. They start 30 to 60 minutes after a dose and subside within a few hours if another dose is not taken (short-duration response). They may affect only a small area, such as the foot or hand, or major segments of the body, such as the limbs on one or both sides. Dyskinesias may involve the whole body, including the trunk. They have a flowing, dancing appearance. The affected limb or portion of the body moves back and forth without any clear pattern. They do not have a truly rhythmic pattern like tremor. Dyskinesias make the person look nervous, but actually those affected deny feeling nervous when experiencing them. These are an uncommon side effect during the first years of DLB or Parkinson's disease.

Dyskinesias represent an excessive levodopa effect. This makes sense in the context of parkinsonism. Recall that too little brain dopamine results in the slowing of body movement. Obviously, too much brain dopamine should result in excessive

movement, and that is exactly the reason for levodopa-induced
dyskinesias. Dyskinesias often involve only one limb or one side
of the body because of the uneven loss of brain dopamine in the
striatum. With administered levodopa, some striatal regions
can have excessive dopamine and others too little.

Note that these dyskinesias are not associated with pain, and
sometimes affected individuals are oblivious to their presence. They
are not dangerous. However, they get in the way if quite prominent.

Dyskinesias Are Usually Easy to Treat

As stated previously, levodopa-induced dyskinesias represent
an excessive response to levodopa and have a short-duration
pattern. Thus reducing the carbidopa/levodopa dosage by a
small amount makes sense. If that strategy proves insufficient,
the dosage can be further lowered once again by a small amount
until the dyskinesias are gone. For example, if one is taking two
and a half tablets three times daily and dyskinesias are problematic, all subsequent doses should be reduced to two tablets,
and, if necessary, to one and a half tablets (three times daily).
However, if the carbidopa/levodopa dose becomes too low,
then parkinsonism can again become problematic, so a happy
medium is desirable. Since dyskinesias obey short-duration
rules, the total daily dose is irrelevant; a carbidopa/levodopa
dose taken yesterday will not influence dyskinesias today.

Dystonia: Not Levodopa-Induced Dyskinesias

Other types of involuntary movements must be distinguished
from levodopa-induced dyskinesias so that the treatment is
appropriate. In DLB, PDD, and Parkinson's disease, dystonia
is common and is a primary symptom of the Lewy disorder,
not due to treatment. Dystonia is an involuntary muscle contraction state, sometimes resembling a cramp. Common dystonias included toes curling or cocked up, inversion of a foot,
or cramp-like pain in the calf. Less commonly, cramp-like

postures in a hand may occur. Dystonias may be painful due to the muscle contraction, much like a simple cramp.

Dystonias in the setting of DLB, PDD, or Parkinson's disease suggest undertreatment with levodopa, rather than an excessive effect. If they are present most of the day, the carbidopa/levodopa doses may be too low. If they come and go, this may point to the levodopa effect wearing off. Sometimes one of the first clues to a declining levodopa response (wearing off; short-duration effect) is dystonic curling of the toes or other limited dystonias. As discussed earlier, this is treated with appropriate shortening of the interval between levodopa doses. Only very rarely is dystonia caused by carbidopa/levodopa.

Tremor Is Not Dyskinesia

Tremor is defined as a regular, repetitive movement. The repeating movements are patterned like a sine-wave from high-school math class. This rhythmic movement contrasts with the chaotic, flowing movements of levodopa-induced dyskinesias. Tremor does not represent an excessive levodopa effect but usually an inadequate amount of levodopa.

Akathisia Is Not Dyskinesia

Akathisia is a medical term implying an inner restlessness, a feeling that one wants to move. This is not experienced by people with levodopa-induced dyskinesias; in fact, many people often feel most relaxed when dyskinesias are present. A feeling of inner nervousness or akathisia typically reflects insufficient levodopa coverage. To observers, those with akathisia appear stiff and slow, or exhibiting parkinsonian. Thus if one feels restless but appears nonmoving (except for tremor), then an insufficient levodopa effect may be present. Conversely, if others notice involuntarily movements but there is no restlessness, then levodopa-induced dyskinesias may be present. This is an important distinction, as the treatment of one is the opposite of the other.

Amantadine for Dyskinesia Treatment?

In the setting of DLB or PDD, levodopa-induced dyskinesias are rarely problematic, since they can be controlled by reducing the carbidopa/levodopa dosage. Perfect control is not necessary, as minor dyskinesias cause no disability (e.g., a wiggling foot when sitting). In rare individuals reduction of carbidopa/levodopa sufficient to abolish dyskinesias is associated with recurrence of intolerable parkinsonism; thus, there is no therapeutic window and either the person is underdosed with parkinsonism or is overdosed with dyskinesias. In this circumstance amantadine may be considered. Amantadine works through a different neurotransmitter system than that for dopamine and tends to reduce dyskinesias without worsening parkinsonism.

As discussed in Chapter 7, amantadine can provoke hallucinations in susceptible individuals. Therefore, it is best avoided in those with DLB or PDD. However, occasional individuals with dyskinesias may need to have amantadine gradually introduced after adjustment of the carbidopa/levodopa dosage.

Amantadine comes in only one size, 100-mg tablets. It may be taken with food or on an empty stomach. For dyskinesias, it may be started with one tablet in the morning. After a week or so, it may be increased to one tablet in the morning and one at lunchtime. Finally, a third dose may be introduced later in the day. There is a dose-related effect and adding a fourth or fifth dose during the waking day is often more effective in abolishing dyskinesias; however, the hallucination potential will be substantially increased with these higher doses. Restated, amantadine is best avoided for treating DLB or PDD, but for refractory levodopa dyskinesias, it can be carefully introduced.

Finally, it should be noted that amantadine has very similar properties to memantine (Namenda), a drug approved for treatment of dementia. Both drugs block a receptor in the brain for the neurotransmitter glutamate (the NMDA receptor). Hence, amantadine and memantine can be additive in their side effects. Memantine may be helpful to a mild extent in treating the dementia of DLB or PDD (addressed in Chapter 12). However, there are rare reports of memantine provoking hallucinations, and predictably, this problem will increase with added amantadine.

SUMMARY

In this chapter we have emphasized that flexibility in dosing is important in managing parkinsonism. As long as one knows the rules about how carbidopa/levodopa works in the body, systematic dosage adjustments can be made, guided by personal observations.

9

Other Levodopa-Responsive Problems

Anxiety, Insomnia, and Pain

Carbidopa/levodopa is well recognized to effectively treat movement ("motor") problems in DLB and PDD, as well as in typical Parkinson's disease. However, symptoms responding to levodopa also include anxiety and insomnia. Moreover, pain control may improve with optimized levodopa dosages. The role for carbidopa/levodopa in treating these symptoms cannot be overemphasized; quality of life may markedly improve with optimized dosage.

ANXIETY

Anxiety is a normal part of the human existence. It is normal to become nervous before a school test or speaking before a large audience. In fact, some of us are especially nervous or anxious as part of our normal makeup. However, newly developing anxiety is a frequent component of DLB, PDD, and Parkinson's disease. In the context of these disorders, anxiety may occasionally be the most troublesome symptom, even bordering on panic. The good news is that this is often treatable with carbidopa/levodopa.

The usual anxiety everyone experiences, or the excessive anxiety of nervous people, does not respond to levodopa. Certain anxiety is normal, such as during family crises and arguments. If a person has been nervous all of their life, levodopa will not be the solution; such anxiety is not due to brain dopamine deficiency. However, anxiety that develops after, or a little before the onset of DLB, PDD, or Parkinson's disease is different. If recently, small issues have provoked panic and this is not a lifelong pattern, levodopa therapy may prove helpful.

The anxiety experienced by those with DLB or PDD may occasionally reach crisis proportions. Emergency room physicians are familiar with older adults being brought in by concerned family members because "mom is in a panic." Sometimes a Valium-like drug is prescribed to establish a quick response. Medications from the Valium class are termed benzodiazepines and include such agents as alprazolam (Xanax), lorazepam (Ativan), clonazepam (Klonopin), as well as Valium itself (diazepam). Benzodiazepines are very sedating, which is beneficial in the emergency room to relax the nervous person; however, ongoing sedation is not acceptable on a long-term basis. Moreover, these drugs contribute to imbalance (fall risk) and tend to impair thinking. Thus, if a benzodiazepine is prescribed for rapid control, there needs to be a different management plan going forward.

Sometimes panicked and confused older adults are administered an antipsychotic drug for rapid control. Nearly all of these antipsychotics (neuroleptics) block dopamine receptors and should not be used in those with DLB or PDD. The list of these drugs is long but includes haloperidol (Haldol), olanzapine (Zyprexa), risperidone (Risperdal), aripiprazole (Abilify), and ziprasidone (Geodon). Generally, most clinicians know that these drugs should not be given to those with DLB, PDD, or Parkinson's disease, so this should not be a issue.

Two drugs from this antipsychotic class are not contraindicated: quetiapine (Seroquel) and clozapine (Clozaril). These may have a role in reducing severe anxiety if other strategies have failed. However, a primary strategy that we will emphasize is an optimized dosage of carbidopa/levodopa.

Carbidopa/Levodopa Treatment of Lewy Body Anxiety

Anxiety developing in the context of DLB, PDD, or Parkinson's disease is often controllable with adequate dosage of carbidopa/levodopa. It may surface due to either insufficient carbidopa/levodopa or as a levodopa wearing-off problem. Each issue will be considered next.

Anxiety is present continuously: insufficient levodopa.

If the person is anxious throughout the day and for no good reason, inadequate levodopa coverage could be responsible. Review Chapter 6 for the carbidopa/levodopa dosage escalation schedule (see Box 6.1). Note that anxiety, like many other levodopa-responsive symptoms, may respond in an all-or-none fashion to carbidopa/levodopa. In other words, low and slightly raised doses may not be beneficial, but once an adequate dosage is reached, the treatment threshold is crossed and anxiety resolves. This may require as much as two and a half to three tablets of 25/100 regular (immediate-release) carbidopa/levodopa for each dose (on am empty stomach).

Anxiety or panic is coming and going: levodopa wearing off.

If anxiousness is absent part of the day but recurring, this may reflect wearing-off of the levodopa effect. Pay attention to the pattern over the day. If wearing-off is the problem, likely the size of the individual dose is adequate but the effect does not last until the time of the next dose. As discussed in Chapter 8, simply reducing the interval between doses to match the response duration is the appropriate strategy (do not lower the amount of individual doses). This will necessitate adding an extra dose or two to provide continuous coverage, and that is appropriate. This may well be necessary at bedtime and during the night (see Insomnia section that follows).

Other Options for Anxiety Failing Levodopa Treatment

If carbidopa/levodopa treatment fails to manage anxiety despite attempts to optimize the dosage, severe anxiety may demand other strategies. This situation then becomes more complicated, and the responses are less predictable. The benzodiazepine drug class cited above (Valium-like medications) often is considered. However, caution is necessary in using this drug class because of their potential to impair balance and cognition or provoke sedation. If these medications are used, they should be used sparingly.

Quetiapine (Seroquel) may be used for treatment of irrational anxiety. Often a single dose at bedtime is helpful or adequate. A morning dose may also be used to quell anxiety, but it is very sedating and not everyone tolerates daytime administration. A common strategy is to start with a single bedtime dose of one-half to one tablet of 25 mg quetiapine at bedtime. It can slowly be raised by 12.5-mg increments, guided by the response. In the setting of DLB or PDD, bedtime doses are usually not raised beyond 150 mg and at most 200 mg, although much higher dosages are used by psychiatrists for other conditions. If anxiousness is very problematic despite this, a morning dose of 12.5 mg can be added. This may prove very sedating but should also have a calming effect. The morning dose can be raised, but in DLB or PDD, it is rarely increased beyond 50 mg. The intent is to calm but not "snow" the person; excessive sleepiness is a limiting side effect of this drug.

Note there is a warning about all the drugs from the quetiapine drug class (both "typical" and "atypical" neuroleptics):

administration to demented patients has been associated with increased mortality. This finding is from studies focusing on statistical risks. The reason for this risk has not been studied, but may relate to chronic oversedation. However, quetiapine does not carry a major mortality risk, and this needs to be balanced against quality of life.

Occasionally, anxiety in this setting responds to a medication from the Prozac class of drugs, which are discussed in more detail in Chapter 18. These are termed selective serotonin reuptake inhibitors (SSRIs) and are routinely used for psychological depression. However, they may help those who are constantly ruminating about something; this may help to break the chain of troublesome thoughts. If such rumination is driving anxiety, one of these medications may be tried.

Anxiety treatment includes environmental strategies, often by trial and error. Familiar surroundings tend to have a calming effect; thus visiting relatives in another city may provoke panic, returning home may do the opposite. Certain music may prove soothing, if properly selected. Quiet voices in the household and avoiding arguments can only be helpful. Finally, the benefits from a good night's sleep cannot be overestimated (see Insomnia section, below).

For prominent anxiety that has failed levodopa treatment, involvement of psychiatry is typically advisable. For severe and very disruptive panic disorders, hospitalization may be an option. An old treatment, electroconvulsive therapy (ECT) is reserved for people with such problems that cannot be treated with simpler measures. Although it may sound barbaric, it has markedly improved the lives of people with uncontrollable panic disorders, seemingly without persistent side effects.

INSOMNIA

Like anxiety, insomnia is common in DLB and PDD. Sleep problems experienced by the general population will not respond to levodopa treatment, whereas insomnia beginning in the context of DLB or Parkinson's disease may respond to carbidopa/levodopa.

The reason insomnia is common in DLB, PDD, and Parkinson's disease often relates to certain parkinsonian symptoms, which include akathisia (restlessness), stiffness (rigidity), tremor, or inability to turn in bed or get comfortable. These and related symptoms are very responsive to levodopa. Carbidopa/levodopa works for insomnia in this setting not because it causes drowsiness, but because it allows people to get comfortable so that natural sleep can ensue.

The long-duration levodopa response (discussed in Chapter 8) relates to the buildup of levodopa benefit with ongoing treatment; it lasts around the clock. For those with insomnia who are just starting carbidopa/levodopa, the daytime doses often effectively treat this via an around-the-clock effect, once the dosage is sufficiently high to be therapeutic (Chapter 6). On the other hand, if the levodopa response comes and goes (wearing off), the daytime doses may not extend into the night, with resulting insomnia. Another dose is then required, but how much and when?

How Much Levodopa?

Whatever dose works best during the waking day is the dose to use for insomnia. A common mistake is to assume that less levodopa is needed at night; however, experience indicates otherwise. The sleep benefit reflects an all-or-nothing response; low dosages will fail to work and only the dosage producing the on response will counter insomnia (i.e., reaching the therapeutic threshold). Thus, if a person is taking two 25/100 tablets three times during the day, then that is the dose to use for insomnia as well.

When to Take It?

If the person is unable to get to sleep, a full dose can be added about an hour before bedtime (it takes up to an hour to kick in).

But I Still Awaken in the Middle of the Night and Can't Return to Sleep!

If the duration of the levodopa beneficial response spans only several hours, it will obviously not continue all night. If it wears off at 3 to 4 A.M., awakening will occur. What should one do if getting back to sleep is impossible? Take another full dose! Have this dose sitting on the nightstand along with a glass of water, ready to take.

What about Sustained-Release Carbidopa/Levodopa (Sinemet CR)?

Theoretically, controlled-release (CR) carbidopa/levodopa should be the answer for those whose bedtime dose of carbidopa/levodopa does not last all night. However, this is often inadequate. Controlled-release carbidopa/levodopa only lasts 60 to 90 minutes longer than regular carbidopa/levodopa. Also, it is more complicated to use as it takes twice as long to kick in (often 2 hours) and does not have a milligram-to-milligram correspondence to regular (immediate-release) carbidopa/levodopa. In fact, a 30 to 50% larger levodopa dose is required when switching to Sinemet CR. Because of this complexity, Sinemet CR will not be addressed further here. It is much simpler and easier to take regular carbidopa/levodopa before bedtime and, if necessary, to repeat a dose at night upon awakening.

PAIN

Pain is a problem for many middle-aged and elderly people in general. It may come from the lower back, arthritic knees, broken bones, or a variety of rheumatologic or other neurologic conditions (e.g., peripheral neuropathy). For those with DLB, PDD, or Parkinson's disease, it is important to recognize that pain from any source is much worse in the setting of inadequate levodopa coverage. Thus too low carbidopa/levodopa doses for a given individual may translate into pain magnification. On the other hand, in the setting of short-duration carbidopa/levodopa responses (wearing off), pain may resolve and then recur with decline of the levodopa effect. The discussion of carbidopa/levodopa dosing in Chapters 6 and 8 is highly relevant to these pain issues. Optimizing the carbidopa/levodopa dosing scheme will help manage pain problems.

But there is more to this pain issue: Lewy disorders (DLB, PDD, Parkinson's disease) sometimes are the primary cause of painful conditions. In Chapter 8, painful muscle contractions and dystonias were discussed. Common dystonias of this type include cramp-like contractions of the toes, feet, or legs (calf). Much less commonly, this occurs in the trunk (e.g., abdomen) or upper limbs. Sciatica-like pain may develop consequent to Lewy disease. One clue to this origin is the waxing and waning of pain with the levodopa response. Pain resolving an hour after a full dose of carbidopa/levodopa but recurring a few hours later is typical. Note that pain resolution requires a full carbidopa/levodopa dose, reflecting the all-or-nothing (threshold) response typical of many levodopa effects.

Rarely, carbidopa/levodopa actually provokes painful dystonias (probably less than 1% of such dystonias). However, this situation will be recognizable by going overnight without carbidopa/levodopa and then taking a full dose in the morning; if the painful contraction occurs 30 to 60 minutes after that carbidopa/levodopa dose and resolves several hours later, then this may reflect such a response.

One should not jump to the conclusion that every instance of pain is due to DLB or PDD. However, if the clinician excludes other causes, this may then be considered. As with other Lewy symptoms, it may be present continuously or may come and go. Optimizing the carbidopa/levodopa coverage as discussed earlier for anxiety is an appropriate strategy.

PROBLEMS CAUSED OR EXACERBATED BY PARKINSON MEDICATIONS

Some problems may be provoked by medications used to replenish brain dopamine and treat parkinsonism. This was the reason for advising simplification of the medication schedule, as discussed in Chapter 7. It is important to recognize such problems so that offending drugs can be targeted for elimination. Medications causing hallucinations and delusions (such as paranoia) and drugs inducing compulsive gambling or other problematic behaviors are discussed in the next two chapters.

10

Hallucinations and Delusions

Defining terms is an appropriate introduction to this chapter.

Hallucinations imply seeing things that are not truly present, or hearing illusory voices or music. In DLB and PDD, hallucinations are nearly always visual and manifest as seeing nonexistent people or objects, such as strangers in the house or yard. The affected individual may realize that he or she is experiencing a hallucination, but some people may not recognize that these are not real. In other disorders auditory hallucinations may be present, such as hearing voices. However, such auditory hallucinations are rare in Lewy disorders.

Delusions are defined as false, often irrational beliefs. Frequently, these will have a theme, such as the conviction that someone is spying, or paranoia about friends or neighbors. A common theme is spousal infidelity, sometimes nonsensical, such as an older adult's accusations of their mate starting an extramarital affair after 50 years of marriage. Capgras syndrome is an uncommon but striking example of delusional thinking in which the spouse or other immediate family member is accused of being an impostor.

Hallucinations or delusions may occur in Parkinson's disease in the absence of frank dementia. However, dementia is the usual setting for these problems. Hallucinations are much more common than delusions. Sometimes they are very limited, perhaps only present at night. Hallucinations are a contraindication to driving a motor vehicle, for obvious reasons.

The fundamental cause of hallucinations and delusions in DLB and PDD is the Lewy neurodegenerative process. The precise region of the brain that is responsible is not known, however.

WHAT MAY PROVOKE HALLUCINATIONS OR DELUSIONS?

These often occur in the absence of any external provocative factors. However, medications are notorious for inciting such problems in susceptible people. Chapter 7 focused on simplifying medications especially for this reason. Drugs for parkinsonism are well-known culprits, in particular two classes: (1) the dopamine agonists: pramipexole (Mirapex), ropinirole (Requip) and rotigotine (Neupro patch); and (2) anticholinergic drugs: trihexyphenidyl (Artane) and benztropine (Cogentin). Carbidopa/levodopa by itself may provoke hallucinations, but that is not very common unless combined with other drugs for parkinsonism.

Prescription pain medications, most notably narcotics (e.g., oxycodone, hydrocodone, oxycontin), may also cause hallucinations or delusions. Anything that is sedating may similarly precipitate such problems, such as drugs from the Valium class (benzodiazepines) or muscle relaxants (cyclobenzaprine, tizanidine). Finally, as we will discuss in Chapter 14, some of the anticholinergic drugs used to dampen bladder urgency may get into the brain and contribute to hallucinations, such as oxybutynin (Ditropan) or tolterodine (Detrol). Most drugs targeting treatment of depression, such as those in the Prozac class (SSRIs), are not likely to cause hallucinations or delusions.

Susceptible people with DLB or PDD may experience hallucinations or delusions provoked by unsuspected infections, such as urinary tract infections. Hence, if hallucinations suddenly surface for no obvious reason, the evaluation should include screening for urinary or other infectious processes.

Impaired nighttime sleep with ongoing sleep deprivation may also contribute to these problems. A good night's sleep on a regular basis can certainly benefit cognition and reduce the potential for hallucinations and delusions. The benefit of carbidopa/levodopa coverage for insomnia, discussed in Chapter 9, is worth reviewing.

Hallucinations or delusions may develop or exacerbate in the setting of daytime drowsiness, which may occur despite apparently adequate nighttime sleep. Daytime sleepiness often indicates poor nighttime sleep quality, as may occur with sleep apnea or periodic movements of sleep. These are treatable conditions and will be discussed in Chapter 16.

MEDICATIONS FOR HALLUCINATIONS AND DELUSIONS

Once contributory factors have been eliminated or minimized, medications can be used to treat hallucinatory or delusional tendencies. Chapter 12 includes discussion of medications for improving memory: donepezil (Aricept) and rivastigmine (Exelon patch). These two drugs may also reduce tendencies toward hallucinations and delusions. They are usually well tolerated and are a reasonable initial treatment strategy. Review Chapter 12 for details about these medications and dosage if hallucinations or delusions are present and require treatment.

Medications that specifically target hallucinations and delusions without worsening parkinsonism are quetiapine and clozapine. Neither of these drugs blocks dopamine receptors, and for this reason they are not contraindicated. Quetiapine (Seroquel) is the drug most commonly used to treat hallucinations and delusions in Lewy disorders; it is usually tolerated. Clozapine has a myriad of side effects, some serious (e.g., a life-threatening drop in the white blood count or other reductions in blood counts). Hence clozapine will not be discussed further in this book.

Quetiapine

This medication was developed to treat schizophrenia and related disorders. For those conditions it is used in high doses and taken twice each day. For hallucinations or delusions due to DLB or PDD it is effective at much lower doses and is typically taken as a single bedtime dose.

Quetiapine is very sedating; thus a single bedtime dose is preferred. Occasional people starting quetiapine will sleep late into the morning and are hard to waken. This situation is not dangerous and often responds to a dosage reduction.

Quetiapine is typically started with either half or a whole 25-mg tablet at bedtime. If the hallucinations or delusions are very troublesome, it may be increased every 3 to 4 days, guided by the response. If the hallucinations or delusions are not too severe, then slowly escalating the dose every week is reasonable. Quetiapine is usually raised by half-tablet increments using the 25-mg tablets—for example, 25 mg, raised to 37.5 mg (one and a half tablets), then 50 mg (two tablets), etc. In most cases, 25 mg to 200 mg as a single bedtime dose is effective; rarely is it necessary to go much higher. If disruptive behavior is evident earlier in the day, a lower dose may be added each morning. Sometimes such a morning dose causes extreme drowsiness, so it should be initiated at 12.5 or 25 mg. To put this into context, dosages for schizophrenia and related disorders are usually several hundred milligrams per day, in contrast to the lower dosages used in DLB and PDD.

The drug class containing quetiapine is classified as atypical neuroleptics. The U.S. Food and Drug Administration has warned that all medications in both the typical and atypical neuroleptic drug classes carry a small risk of increased mortality.

The reason for this risk has not been established. Neurologists prescribing quetiapine for these problems have generally not found it necessary to restrict use of quetiapine. It serves a very useful purpose, and benefits appear to offset the small risks.

SUMMARY: RECIPE FOR TREATMENT

There is a logical order for dealing with these hallucinations or delusions if the cause is not immediately apparent. This begins with assessment by the primary clinician:

1. Review the medication list for drugs that may enter the brain and cause problems. Minor drugs for parkinsonism may be tapered off, one by one, if this has not already been done (Chapter 7).
2. Address whether there is some other active medical problem, such as a urinary tract infection or pneumonia.
3. Treat sleep disorders.
4. Consider using either donepezil or rivastigmine (dosing is outlined in Chapter 12).
5. If the delusions or hallucinations are still uncontrolled, start a bedtime dose of quetiapine.
6. Adjust the quetiapine dose upward, guided by the response.
7. Rarely a small reduction of carbidopa/levodopa may be necessary.

11

Pathologic Behaviors Provoked by Dopamine Agonist Drugs

Gambling, Sex, Eating, and Spending

Dopamine agonists are synthetic medications that stimulate dopamine receptors. They are commonly used for treatment of Parkinson's disease and in lower doses for restless legs syndrome. This drug class includes pramipexole (Mirapex), ropinirole (Requip), and the rotigotine patch (Neupro). These drugs have special properties, with unique adverse effects that are not intuitively associated with the drug. Hence, a brief chapter is devoted to these side effects. If the patient is not taking one of these medications, this chapter may be skipped.

THE PROBLEM

Several years ago clinicians recognized that pramipexole and ropinirole were associated with the development of pathologic

117

gambling. Insidiously, a minority of people who were prescribed these medications began experiencing the desire to gamble, such as at casinos or online. For some, this was an exacerbation of prior tendencies, but for others this desire came out of the blue, with no prior gambling history. Other types of compulsive pathologic behaviors soon were also recognized in some people treated with these drugs. This included inappropriate hypersexual behavior (extramarital affairs, pornography) and compulsive spending, eating, drinking, or smoking. In many people, this behavior was completely out of character. The common element was the initiation of pramipexole or ropinirole. The behaviors did not develop immediately, but insidiously became apparent after the medication was slowly escalated into the therapeutic range. Patients and family were often oblivious to the behavior or relation to the drug until specifically asked about it in the doctor's office.

The common theme among these compulsive behaviors is that they are inherently rewarding human experiences. It became recognized that use of these dopamine agonist drugs by some people was associated with a pathologic drive to excessively engage in such activities as gambling, sex, eating, or spending. For affected people, this began to dominate their thoughts and actions.

Who would think that a drug could drive specific hedonistic or rewarding behaviors? Experience in the clinic and published evidence, however, corroborates this risk. The two primary agents that have been implicated are pramipexole (Mirapex) and ropinirole (Requip). The rotigotine patch has also been associated with such behaviors, but apparently less frequently. Rotigotine pharmacology is very similar to that of pramipexole and ropinirole, indicating that it may have similar potential. However, it is usually administered in lower doses and thus may be less likely to elicit these problems. Rotigotine has not been available in the United States for the past few years.

HOW TO RECOGNIZE PATHOLOGIC BEHAVIORS

We all have some bad habits and not everything can be blamed on the medications. Just because someone lost money at the casino or accessed a pornography Web site does not mean that a dopamine agonist drug was the reason.

Dopamine agonist–related behavioral disorders develop insidiously. They do not suddenly surface when one of these drugs is started or the dosage is raised. People experiencing this problem are often oblivious to the development and progression of these behaviors. Typically, it is the spouse or a family member that notices a major character change. The need to travel to a casino, compulsively buy lotto or pull-tab tickets, or gamble online starts to dominate the person's life. In others, sexual ideation becomes the dominant theme, which is much more likely among men; they may uncharacteristically demand sex many times a day (often with failed erections) or sneak off to view online pornography Web sites. Compulsive spending is problematic in others, such as purchasing many of the same devices or clothing (e.g., DVD players, TVs, shoes or watches). Compulsive occupation with food and eating may lead to weight gain. In fact, anything that is inherently rewarding can become a focus among those with dopamine agonist–elicited behavioral syndromes.

An objective opinion and treatment instructions from the clinician are crucial if this is suspected. Since the affected person may have poor insight into this pattern of behavior, spouses and family should avoid a confrontation; let the clinician be the arbiter and then organize the treatment plan. Family members and spouses should be present to contribute to the discussion, as the affected person often tends to minimize what is becoming a major problem.

WHO IS AT RISK?

Through clinical experience at the Mayo Clinic, it has become clear that the offending drugs have unique pharmacologic properties: they bind with high affinity to one specific type of dopamine receptor, the dopamine D3 receptor (see below). Although predisposing characteristics have been proposed, the affected people seen in the Mayo Neurology Clinic often have no predictive background characteristics.

In our PD-DLB clinic, this problem has been associated only with higher doses of the specific dopamine agonist drugs. For treatment of Parkinson's disease, higher doses are necessary in order to obtain a therapeutic effect. An exception to this observation, however, is that clinicians in the Mayo Sleep Center have documented such problematic behaviors in several people taking only low doses of pramipexole or ropinirole for restless legs syndrome.

WHY OR HOW WOULD A DRUG INDUCE PATHOLOGIC BEHAVIORS?

The answer to this question is found in the unique pharmacology of the implicated dopamine agonist drugs. By definition, dopamine agonists bind to dopamine receptors. Pramipexole, ropinirole, and rotigotine do not have strong affinity for all five types of dopamine receptors, but rather have specific affinity for the dopamine D3 receptor. In contrast, the natural substance, levodopa is transformed into dopamine that binds to all the brain dopamine receptors, D1 through D5. So why should drugs that activate the specific D3 receptor induce such behaviors? In fact, the D3 receptor is the perfect candidate for this problem. It is well recognized that dopamine D3 receptors are largely localized to the brain's limbic system. Among other things, the limbic system is known to be the brain's hedonistic center, thought to mediate primal rewarding behaviors.

TREATMENT

In Chapter 5, we advised avoiding these dopamine agonist drugs in the context of DLB or PDD, primarily because of their potential for inducing hallucinations or delusions. However, occasional people with DLB are started on a dopamine agonist, and sometimes those with PDD have been on them for years, predating the dementia. Hence, this chapter may be relevant to some patients.

Experience has taught us that when these problematic behaviors surface, the dopamine agonist drug needs to be tapered off. Dose reductions have not been sufficient for treating this condition. Psychiatric medications for these behavioral problems typically fail, as do psychotherapeutic strategies, unless combined with elimination of the agonist drug. Hence, the dopamine agonist medication typically needs to be tapered off in order to stop the problematic behavior.

Detailed drug-tapering strategies were discussed in Chapter 7. The clinician should provide the patient with specific instructions about how to do this.

The response to eliminating the dopamine agonist may not be immediate; it is important to be aware of this. It may take days, weeks, or even months for this compulsive behavioral syndrome to abate. In the meantime, the patient, family, and spouse may need to organize their lives in order to reduce exposure to the risks.

If the dopamine agonist is being used in low doses to treat restless legs syndrome, a drug with different properties will need to be substituted if pathologic behaviors develop. This treatment is discussed in Chapter 16.

If the dopamine agonist is the only drug being used to treat parkinsonism, then carbidopa/levodopa will likely need to be added at some future time. Usually it is wise to defer starting it until the problematic behavior has fully resolved. Carbidopa/levodopa initiation and adjustment are addressed in Chapters 6.

For those with DLB or PDD, it should be possible to eventually eliminate the agonist altogether, which is typically necessary to treat this problem. However, in a small percentage of people, tapering off a dopamine agonist drug will provoke withdrawal symptoms. This might include anxiety, depression, insomnia, agitation, or a variety of other unpleasant experiences. If symptoms of withdrawal begin to surface, a much slower tapering of the dose is appropriate. Ultimately, if the dopamine agonist cannot be stopped, it should be reduced to as low a dose as tolerated. Carbidopa/levodopa can then be added or raised to control the parkinsonism.

It is not clear how to treat the residual pathologic compulsive behaviors that remain while the patient is on the agonist drug. A psychiatrist or psychologist may prove helpful in this setting.

COGNITIVE PROBLEMS

A central feature of DLB and PDD is cognitive impairment. Cognition refers to memory, thinking, judgment, and higher-level thought. It includes subtle components such as task organization and prioritizing, multitasking, or finding our way home in an unfamiliar locality. Enhancing cognition in the face of Lewy disease is the focus of the chapter in this section.

12

Dementia

Impaired Thinking and Judgment; Confusion

Dementia implies problems with cognition (thinking), and this is a fundamental component of DLB and PDD. Dementia also implies that the cognitive problems are sufficiently troublesome to affect activities of daily living. Less severe impairment of memory or thinking that does not interfere with daily activities is classified as mild cognitive impairment (MCI). MCI may be a prelude to dementia. If MCI accompanies parkinsonism, then the treatment strategies outlined in this text are appropriate.

Dementia does not necessarily mean that a rapid progression to an advanced state is inevitable. Dementia may be relatively mild and well compensated, especially with the help of the spouse and family; it may remain that way for years.

The cognitive profile of DLB and PDD was described in Chapter 4. To review, this impairment affects several major components of intellect. This includes executive function, localized to the frontal lobes of the brain. Visuospatial conceptualization is similarly affected, which reflects problems in the posterior brain (i.e., parietal and occipital lobes). Memory declines in DLB and PDD, but less than in Alzheimer's disease.

Fluctuations in mental clarity are often noted in these Lewy disorders, where near-normal thinking may be followed hours later by confusion.

In Chapter 4, the process of diagnosing DLB and PDD was also discussed. Before clinicians consider such a diagnosis, however, they must be certain that they have not overlooked any other treatable causes or contributors. Sometimes the DLB or PDD diagnosis is correct but the dementia is exacerbated by some other factor. In this chapter, those factors and the appropriate workup are considered.

THE SEARCH FOR TREATABLE CAUSES

One should not arrive at the final diagnosis of a neurodegenerative dementia before considering treatable factors, including medical conditions, brain lesions (e.g., bleeds), and medication effects. This is especially relevant if there has been a rapid decline or recent onset.

Review of the Medication List

Prescription drugs are a common cause of cognitive impairment. Before ordering tests, it is appropriate to go over all medications that the patient is taking. Commonly prescribed drugs that can impair cognition include those shown in Table 12.1. This is not an exhaustive list. The primary clinician should decide what, if any, medication should be eliminated.

Tests for Other Causes

There are no specific tests for DLB, PDD, or Parkinson's disease. However, when cognition is impaired, clinicians need to consider alternative causes or contributing factors. Testing varies with the clinical features and might include the following tests.

Table 12.1 Commonly Prescribed Medications that Can Impair Thinking and Memory*

Narcotic Pain Medications	Non-narcotic Pain Medications	Muscle Relaxants	Anxiety Relievers	Tricyclic Drugs for Depression	Drugs for Overactive Bladder	Drugs for Irritable Bowel	Parkinsonism Drugs
Oxycodone (in Percodan, Oxycontin); hydrocodone (in Vicodin, Lortab); codeine (in Tylenol #3 and others)	Tramadol (Ultram, Ultracet); butalbital (in headache medications)	Tizanidine (Zanaflex); baclofen (Lioresal); cyclobenzaprine (Flexeril); orphenadrine (Norgesic, Norflex); carisoprodol (Soma); chlorzoxazone (Parafon Forte)	Benzodiazepines: clonazepam (Klonopin); diazepam (Valium); alprazolam (Xanax); lorazepam (Ativan); clorazepate (Tranxene). Hydroxyzine (Atarax, Vistaril)	Amitriptyline (Elavil); nortriptyline (Pamelor); desipramine (Norpramine); imipramine (Tofranil); doxepin (Sinequan); trimipramine (Surmontil)	Tolterodine (Detrol); oxybutynin (Ditropan, Oxytrol); darifenacin (Enablex); hyoscyamine (Cystospaz, Levsin, Levsinex); solifenacin (Vesicare); fesoterodine (Toviaz)	Dicyclomine (Bentyl); hyoscyamine; atropine; scopolamine; propantheline (Pro-Banthine); clidinium (ingredient in Librax)	Ttrihexyphenidyl (Artane); benztropine (Cogentin); procyclidine (Kemadrin); biperiden (Akineton)

* Note that sleep aids, including over-the-counter diphenhydramine, can contribute to nighttime confusion when taken at bedtime.

Bran scan.

Brain tumors, strokes, bleeds, or other brain lesions, as well as hydrocephalus (normal pressure hydrocephalus [NPH]), can be assessed with a brain scan; this might be either computed tomography (CT) or magnetic resonance imaging (MRI). An MRI scan provides much higher resolution, but a CT brain may be sufficient for identifying structural lesions affecting brain function. Note that MRI scans cannot easily be done in those with pacemakers, deep brain stimulation devices, other metal (e.g., shrapnel) or wires in their body (artificial joints are acceptable).

Blood work.

General medical conditions such as liver failure, thyroid insufficiency, or other major medical problems may secondarily impair brain function. To assess for such conditions simple blood tests are done: complete blood count, comprehensive chemistry panel, vitamin B12 level, thyroid function, plus whatever else is suggested by the history.

Urinalysis.

In susceptible people something as simple as an untreated urinary tract infection may lead to cognitive decompensation.

Pursuit of medical symptoms as appropriate.

Concurrent medical conditions with major symptoms such as marked weight loss, severe lethargy, or shortness of breath raise concern that the cognitive impairment might be part of a more general medical condition (e.g., occult cancer). This should be addressed by the primary care physician.

Spinal fluid examination (cerebrospinal fluid [CSF]).

A CSF examination is not necessary in every case of dementia. The purpose of a CSF examination is to pursue possible infectious or immune-mediated causes of brain dysfunction. If the history suggests that this is unlikely, the clinician may then decide against performing a CSF examination. However, there are occasional patients in whom a chronic, insidious infection might be causative, such as Lyme disease, syphilis, or chronic meningitis. Similarly, an immune-mediated disorder might target the brain and only be diagnosed with the aid of a CSF examination. Examples of such immunologic conditions include lupus, sarcoidosis, or remote immunologic effects triggered by cancer (paraneoplastic). The CSF examination may not always identify the cause, but if the results are abnormal, this finding would signal a search for an infectious or inflammatory process.

Address sleep disorders.

Impaired nighttime sleep may affect daytime mental clarity. Notorious for doing this is sleep apnea, discussed in detail in Chapter 16. Overnight oximetry is a simple screening method for detecting sleep apnea (although it is not 100% conclusive). A clue that a sleep disorder is contributing to impaired thinking is daytime drowsiness.

Formal psychometrics.

Formal testing of intellectual function is performed by a psychologist. The profile of cognitive problems may help the neurologist determine the diagnosis, although it is not always necessary. Formal psychometric testing may have other utilities in certain situations. For example, such testing may be invaluable in the assessment of pseudo-dementia in which severe depression is the primary reason for the cognitive impairment. It also has other practical benefits, such as providing the health care team insight into whether assistance is needed for management of banking, bill-paying, investments, and other financial matters. The measurement of dementia severity and the cognitive profile may help the clinician select the appropriate medication, which is discussed next.

MEDICATIONS FOR COGNITION

The drugs used to enhance memory and thinking are rather modest in their effects. However, they are often worth trying and are relatively easy to use.

Acetylcholinesterase Inhibitors

Acetylcholine is a brain signaling molecule (neurotransmitter). It has been recognized for decades as being crucial to memory. In animal studies, blocking this neurotransmitter with drugs (anticholinergics) impairs memory, whereas drugs than enhance acetylcholine levels improve memory. Although there are multiple regions in the brain that use acetylcholine as a neurotransmitter, one particular region is thought to be very important to memory, the nucleus basalis, illustrated in Figure 12.1. The neurons in this nucleus have widespread projections to the cortex.

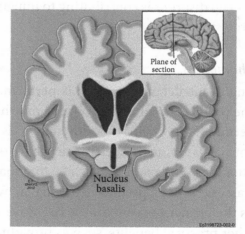

Figure 12.1 The nucleus basalis degenerates in DLB and PDD. It uses acetylcholine as the neurotransmitter, projecting to wide regions of the cortex. Acetylcholine deficiency is associated with memory impairment.

The nucleus basalis degenerates in DLB and PDD. It is assumed that this loss, and the reduction of acetylcholine neurotransmission, contributes to the dementia. Conversely, it makes sense that drugs enhancing acetylcholine neurotransmission might benefit those with DLB and PDD.

The most direct pharmacologic strategy for enhancing brain acetylcholine is via drugs that block the enzyme, acetylcholinesterase. Acetylcholinesterase breaks down acetylcholine, preventing excessive accumulation of this neurotransmitter.

Blocking the enzyme acetylcholinesterase increases brain acetylcholine levels and potentially improves memory. In practice, medications that block this enzyme do improve memory, although the memory enhancement is not dramatic. These drugs also tend to reduce hallucinations and delusions and may be used for that purpose. They have become a standard of treatment for DLB and PDD, although the benefits are limited. Side effects include nausea and stomach cramps. Rarely, diarrhea or worsened tremor may occur.

There are several medications in this class, including donepezil (Aricept), rivastigmine (Exelon), and galantamine (Razadyne). Donepezil and galantamine are administered as a pill. Rivastigmine is primarily used as a patch but is also available in capsule form and oral solution (rivastigmine administered orally is more likely to cause nausea and vomiting than the patch). These drugs are not used in combination. The other medication from this class is tacrine (Cognex), which is infrequently prescribed because of its potential for liver toxicity.

It is not proven that any one of these medications is more efficacious than the other when full dosages are used. The primary differences relate to gastrointestinal side effects, which appear least with oral donepezil and the rivastigmine patch.

Donepezil (Aricept).
Donepezil is typically started as a single 5 mg tablet taken once daily, usually in the morning, but it can be taken at bedtime.

After an interval, such as 6 weeks, it is then raised to two tablets once daily. I usually recommend maintaining this dosage (10 mg daily) for an additional 6 weeks and then deciding whether it is beneficial; if not, it can be discontinued. Some clinicians will also try dose escalation to 15 mg (three tablets) once daily. Recently, a 23 mg pill was made available. However, there is insufficient evidence to show that it has meaningful benefits beyond the 10 to 15 mg daily dose. This 23 mg size is more likely to cause gastrointestinal side effects.

Rivastigmine patch (Exelon).

Rivastigmine is better tolerated in patch-form than the capsules or oral solution. The patch is the formulation usually employed. The capsules and oral solution are more likely to cause nausea and vomiting. The patch comes in two sizes: 4.6 mg/24 hours and 9.5 mg/24 hours. Therapy is started with the smaller size (4.6 mg/24 hours). It is applied once every 24 hours. It should be placed on skin that is neither wet nor irritated. The patch is generally applied on the trunk or back and placement should be in different spots so that the same spot is not reused within 2 weeks. After 4 to 6 weeks it can be changed to the larger size, 9.5 mg/24 hours. After another 4 to 6 weeks it can be stopped if there is no benefit.

Skin irritation is a potential side effect and the reason for rotating the placement site. Like the other acetylcholinesterase inhibitor drugs, it may be discontinued if it is not beneficial. A slightly larger rivastigmine dose in patch form (13.3 mg/24 hours) should become available in the near future.

Rivastigmine capsules (Exelon).

Oral rivastigmine capsules are typically started with a single 1.5 mg capsule twice daily, with meals. Nausea or other gastrointestinal symptoms may limit use of oral rivastigmine, and the dosage is raised slowly to limit such side effects. If tolerated, it can be raised every 2 weeks from 1.5 mg twice daily to 3 mg, then 4.5 mg, then 6 mg twice daily. It is available in the following sizes: 1.5, 3, 4.5, and 6 mg capsules.

Rivastigmine oral solution (Exelon).

The oral solution comes in 120 mL bottles with 2 mg of rivastigmine per milliliter. It may be stored at room temperature but should not be frozen. The standard 4 ounce bottle is supplied with a syringe for proper dosing, plus an instruction sheet. The syringe allows for a maximum amount of 3 mL, which is 6 mg. It may be swallowed directly or mixed with juice or soda pop. The oral solution allows for more graduated dose escalation, which may be helpful for those who are easily nauseated. Conventionally, it is started with 1.5 mg (1.5 mL) twice daily (with meals) and slowly raised. If tolerated, the dosage may be raised every 2 weeks with the same increments as listed above for the capsules, up to 6 mg twice daily.

Galantamine (Razadyne).

This comes in two pill formulations, regular (plus an oral solution) and extended-release. The regular formulation is started with one 4 mg tablet twice daily for a month, then one 8 mg tablet twice daily for a month, then one 12 mg tablet twice daily. After an additional 4 to 6 weeks it can be stopped or tapered off if there is no benefit. The oral solution is dosed similarly. The 8 mg extended-release capsule is taken once each morning for a month, then switched to the 16 mg capsule taken once daily for a month, and finally the 24 mg capsule taken once each morning. After 4 to 6 weeks on this highest dose it can be discontinued if there is no benefit.

Note that these acetylcholinesterase inhibitor drugs, which enhance acetylcholine transmission, work opposite a class of bladder drugs. Anticholinergic medications that reduce bladder hyperactivity block acetylcholine receptors (see Table 12.1). Most of the drugs targeting the bladder are also capable of getting into the brain. Thus it is not rational to use these two competing drugs classes at the same time. The single bladder drug that is acceptable is trospium (Sanctura), which has a chemical configuration that prevents it from crossing the blood–brain barrier.

NMDA (Glutamate) Inhibitor: Memantine (Namenda)

Memantine was FDA approved for Alzheimer's disease, but it may be tried for DLB or PDD. There is one report of hallucinations, which is not surprising since its properties are very similar to those of amantadine; amantadine may provoke hallucinations in Lewy disorders, as discussed in Chapter 7. Memantine may be used concurrently with the acetylcholinesterase inhibitor drugs discussed above. The mechanism of memantine action is blocking of the neurotransmitter glutamate, a very common brain signaling molecule. Memantine blocks only one type of glutamate receptor (NMDA).

Memantine comes in both a regular tablet and an extended-release capsule. Patients using the regular tablet should start with one 5 mg tablet once daily for a week, then take one 5 mg tablet twice daily. A week later one of the two doses can be raised to two 5 mg tablets, and a week after that both doses can be raised to 10 mg twice daily. This is the maximum dosage. If there is no benefit after a few weeks it can be tapered off. The oral solution is similarly escalated.

The extended-release capsule comes in 7 mg, 14 mg, 21 mg, and 28 mg sizes. The simplest strategy is to take a single 7 mg capsule once each morning for 1 week, then two capsules (14 mg) once daily the next week, then three capsules (21 mg) daily the next week, and then ultimately 28 mg (i.e., four 7 mg capsules) once daily, which is the maximum dosage. The dosage should not be increased if there are substantial side effects, which might include dizziness, loose stools, or headache. If hallucinations begin after starting memantine, it should probably be tapered off.

Dopamine and Cognition

What should not be overlooked in the setting of DLB and PDD is that dopamine deficiencies may make at least a small contribution to the associated cognitive problems. The slowed movement (bradykinesia) of parkinsonism is paralleled by slowed thinking, termed bradyphrenia. Attention may be impaired by the inner discomfort and inner restlessness (akathisia) of Lewy disorders. Slower processing and impaired attention may benefit from carbidopa/levodopa therapy; however, it will not substantially improve the primary cognitive deficits.

Depression

Attention may also be impaired by depression, which occurs frequently in DLB and PDD. Treatment of the depression (see Chapter 18) may also improve cognition, albeit modestly in most cases.

Non-Drug Treatment Strategies

Confusion is increased by being in unfamiliar environments. Hence people with cognitive impairment do best in their familiar home environment and with structured activities. Limiting novelty is often helpful and can reduce disorientation.

As discussed earlier, adequate sleep is important for mental clarity. Thus any sleep disorder should be treated. Occasionally, poor sleep habits translate into inadequate sleep time. Some people habitually go to bed very late or set the alarm to arise too early. For most of us, at least 7 hours of good sleep is necessary each night; for many people 8 or even 9 hours is ideal. A clue to inadequate sleep at night is frequent napping during the day or easily falling asleep when reading or watching television. Sleep is addressed in greater detail in Chapters 9 and 16.

Restrictions

If cognition is impaired, it is wise to consider whether certain restrictions are necessary. These may be difficult for the family to impose, and it is often necessary for the clinician to weigh in on this issue to avoid family arguments.

For individuals with impaired cognition, driving usually needs to be limited or discontinued. Judgment is obviously an important component of driving skills, and if it has declined, then driving a car may be dangerous for the driver as well as others on the road. Limitations and restrictions on driving translate into major life changes, and alternative means of transportation will be important.

Management of finances and investments will likely need to be considered at some juncture among people with DLB or PDD. The person's judgment may no longer be sufficient to make sound business decisions. The nature of Lewy dementia is that it affects executive functions, and this may translate into impulsiveness or poor attention to detail. This may be a situation where a formal cognitive assessment (psychometric testing) by a trained psychologist may help advise the patient and family.

Aggression and Acting out

Aggressive or inappropriate behavior is not an expected consequence of Lewy disorders, but it can occur with any dementing illness. Sometimes there are simple reasons for such behavior, such as pain or fear.

If this type of behavioral problem occurs, an appropriate first treatment step is to address situational factors. Is some simple need not being met, such as thirst, hunger, or pain control? Is irritability being exacerbated by impaired sleep? Is there something new in the living situation that is threatening or confusing? Recall that familiar things tend to be calming. It is important to focus on environmental factors that can be modified.

Medications may ultimately be prescribed when simpler strategies are not working. There are no FDA-approved drugs specifically for this purpose. Tranquilizing medications from the Valium class (benzodiazepines) are often used in this setting, but they may add to the person's confusion and can occasionally have a paradoxical effect (worsening symptoms rather than resolving them). These medications should be used sparingly or, not at all. Shorter-acting drugs of this type, such as alprazolam or lorazepam, are preferable to long-acting drugs, if used.

For problems of this type, the medication quetiapine (Seroquel) is usually chosen. It is often prescribed as a single bedtime dose, similar to the dosing strategy discussed for hallucinations and delusions in Chapter 10. This is initiated with a half or whole 25 mg tablet. However, because of its sedating properties, a low dose may also be given early in the day for more immediate effects. Low daytime doses on the order of 12.5 or 25 mg are helpful for producing a calming effect. Despite the sedating properties, quetiapine appears much less likely to induce paradoxical agitation than the Valium class of drugs.

For behavioral stabilization, the bedtime dose of quetiapine may gradually be raised, using the strategy described in Chapter 10 for control of hallucinations (12.5 mg increments, every few days, guided by the response). A dose early in the day usually should be avoided because of sedation; however, the sedating effect may be useful in some circumstances for a calming effect. In that setting, the daytime dose is increased by 12.5 mg increments (half of a 25 mg tablet), guided by the response.

The FDA has mandated a warning about all drugs from the quetiapine class, relating to increased mortality risk. However, with judicious use this risk appears to be very low. It is more than offset by the benefits when these drugs are used appropriately.

Antidepressants from the Prozac class (SSRIs) are sometimes advocated for treating these behavioral problems. Be aware that these are slow to take effect, and benefits may be delayed for weeks. Moreover, they are not consistently effective for behavioral control problems. They do have few side effects.

As discussed in Chapter 11, the dopamine agonist drugs can provoke hypersexual behavior. Sometimes those affected can be quite aggressive in their sexual advances. If that behavior is recognized, the offending dopamine agonist drug should be tapered off.

DYSAUTONOMIA: BLOOD PRESSURE, BLADDER, BOWELS

DLB, PDD, and Parkinson's disease affect the autonomic nervous system. The autonomic nervous system regulates the bowels, bladder, sweating, heart rate, and blood pressure. This regulation is outside of conscious awareness (unless it malfunctions, causing symptoms).

The autonomic nervous system consists of a network of nerve cells and their connections, distributed throughout the body and linked to the central nervous system (brain, spinal cord). This autonomic nervous system mediates many unconscious reflexes such as sweating when hot, or the urge to have a bowel movement when the colon is filled with feces.

The autonomic nervous system is affected by the Lewy neurodegenerative process. It appears that this occurs early in the course of a Lewy disorder. Affected neurons of the autonomic nervous system contain microscopic Lewy bodies, just like affected brain cells.

Constipation and bladder problems are common in DLB, PDD, and Parkinson's disease, reflecting autonomic dysfunction. The most troublesome condition, however, is a drop in blood pressure when standing. This does not occur in everyone with a Lewy disorder but is frequently encountered. The drop in upright blood pressure can result in fainting or near-faints. This condition is termed orthostatic hypotension and will be addressed first in this section.

13

Blood Pressure and Orthostatic Hypotension

Faints, Near-Faints, and Lightheadedness

Case example: Mrs. H. feels lightheaded intermittently during the day. This happens exclusively when she is up and about. Sometimes she notes graying of vision with these episodes. The feeling is not spinning (i.e., not vertigo). She has fainted twice when standing in line at the grocery store. If she sits, she feels much better. It is worse in the morning but may recur any time of the day. She feels fine while lying in bed at night.

Older adults often worry about high blood pressure (BP), yet the opposite problem, low BP, is common among those with DLB or PDD. This is because the Lewy neurodegenerative process impairs the autonomic nervous system. The specific condition that may afflict those with DLB or PDD is *orthostatic hypotension*.

The term *orthostatic* implies the upright position (i.e., standing); *hypotension* translates into low BP. Thus, the low BP occurring in these Lewy disorders develops in the upright position; conversely, it is normal or even high when lying down. When standing or walking, the BP may drop so low that fainting occurs. Among people with orthostatic hypotension, the BP is normal when sitting, although in severe cases, even the sitting BP is low.

Whereas most people with DLB or PDD do not experience symptoms of orthostatic hypotension, it is sufficiently frequent to deserve attention. It often goes undiagnosed, even when fainting occurs. Unrecognized orthostatic hypotension may limit activities and impair the person's quality of life.

The first half of this chapter provides further background, with focus on BP measurement and recognition of orthostatic hypotension. The last half addresses treatment.

NORMALLY, BLOOD PRESSURE IS THE SAME REGARDLESS OF BODY POSITION

The normal autonomic nervous system senses the position of our body with respect to the pull of gravity. It is able to reflexively counter gravity's downward pull on the blood volume when standing (gravity tends to draw blood toward our feet when standing). An important mechanism for countering gravity's pull is the constriction of blood vessel diameter in the lower half of the body. These vessels reflexively constrict during standing, in effect forcing blood up to the brain. The autonomic nervous system mediates these and other reflexive changes to stabilize BP.

Theoretically, our body's aggregate blood vessel system can be thought of as a partially filled column of fluid. The top of the column would be analogous to the brain, and the bottom, the feet. If this column is upright, the fluid is pulled downward by gravity to the bottom of the column (the feet). Extending this analogy, assume that the lower half of the column is able to constrict, narrowing the diameter. If the column is upright, the fluid in the column would then be squeezed to the top (brain) by the constriction, offsetting gravity. This is what happens to the circulation with changes in body position. Blood vessels have muscles in their walls. When the autonomic nervous system senses gravity pulling blood to the lower half of the body, these blood vessel muscles in the lower body constrict, and the BP in the upper half of the body is maintained.

Other reflexive changes also occur, such as changes in the heart rate or strength of the heart's contraction. With such autonomic reflexes, normal people have a stable BP that does not substantially change whether lying, sitting, or standing.

ORTHOSTATIC HYPOTENSION

Individuals with orthostatic hypotension due to DLB or PDD experience faintness with standing because the autonomic nervous system malfunctions. The internal reflexes normally triggered by body position are poorly activated. Thus, the expected compensatory changes in blood vessel diameter and heart beat do not offset the pull of gravity on blood volume. This is the reason for orthostatic hypotension.

Those with DLB and PDD are at risk for orthostatic hypotension not only because of autonomic dysfunction but also because of certain medications. This includes drugs for parkinsonism as well as drugs for other purposes. This recognition is important for treatment, as we will address later in this chapter.

A very low BP results in faints or near-faints. With reduced BP that is not quite that low, the symptoms may not be recognized as being caused by hypotension. Such symptoms includes lightheadedness, fatigue, fogginess, or impaired mental clarity. Note that vertigo, which represents a spinning sensation in the head, is not a symptom of hypotension, but rather is typical of inner-ear dysfunction.

Reductions in BP going from sitting to standing can be substantial and yet not cause symptoms, provided that the standing

BP does not drop below certain values. In other words, the symptoms of low BP (e.g., lightheadedness) are triggered when the standing BP drops below a certain level. The size of the drop per se is not a factor in these symptoms; rather, it is the absolute BP when standing. This recognition helps us treat this problem, since we can specify a standing BP as the minimum to accept and as a treatment target.

BP Measurements and Values of Concern

As discussed in Chapter 6, BP readings are given in two numbers, the systolic (upper number) and the diastolic (lower number). Thus a BP reading of 120/80 contains the systolic value of 120 and the diastolic reading of 80. In healthy people these two values tend to run parallel to each other. In practice, using just the systolic BP to set parameters should be sufficient; this is the approach we will take in this book.

BP readings are specified as millimeters of mercury (mm Hg). This relates to older BP devices that used columns of mercury as a standard of pressure measurement. An applied force elevated mercury in a glass column against gravity; the height of the elevation was in proportion to the applied force. Thus, a systolic value of 120 relates to 120 mm of mercury-column elevation. This is conventionally written as 120 mm Hg. In this book, we will not use the unit "mm Hg" and will give BP readings only as numbers. The systolic BP will be our benchmark when considering orthostatic hypotension. Hence, for the BP reading 120/80, we will ignore the diastolic number and simply use "120."

When is the BP too low? The answer is 90 (systolic). If the standing systolic BP is always over 90, symptoms (lightheadedness, faintness) should not occur. That is not to imply that systolic values below 90 always cause symptoms. However, 90 is a good treatment target; maintaining the systolic BP over that value is recommended.

Most people are unaware of the utility of checking the BP in the standing position. For those with DLB or PDD, standing BP readings should be included with the routine sitting readings.

Symptoms of faintness should make one suspicious of low BP. The BP should be checked while the patient is in the position of faintness (i.e., standing, unless continued standing would lead to a faint). Among those with orthostatic hypotension, the BP typically normalizes when sitting.

If there is any suspicion of orthostatic hypotension, it is wise for the patient to purchase a BP measurement device. Moreover, it should be one that is calibrated into low ranges. Some less expensive devices focus on normal to high BP values, whereas low values simply trigger an "error" reading.

Many people with DLB or PDD do not experience problems with orthostatic hypotension. If a person's BP readings have never been low (e.g., systolic BP always over 120) and there are no symptoms of lightheadedness, an occasional standing BP measurement is sufficient.

Dysfunction of the autonomic nervous system is the primary substrate for low BP problems in DLB and PDD. However, medications often play a major contributory role.

Carbidopa/Levodopa Provokes Orthostatic Hypotension

All drugs for treating parkinsonism potentially exacerbate orthostatic hypotension. They do this roughly in proportion to their capacity to improve parkinsonism. In this book, we have advised those with DLB or PDD to limit these parkinsonism drugs to carbidopa/levodopa. This is the most potent of all the parkinsonism agents, but it is also the most likely to provoke orthostatic hypotension. Considering this in detail will help work around this problem in susceptible people.

The tendency to lower the standing BP is in proportion to the size of the individual carbidopa/levodopa doses; thus, a dose of two carbidopa/levodopa tablets will be more likely to provoke orthostatic hypotension than one tablet. Note that if the doses are spaced sufficiently far apart, the number of tablets per day is not relevant. That is because the tendency to lower the standing BP only lasts for a few hours after each dose.

The specific dynamics of the BP-lowering potential of carbidopa/levodopa are important to recognize. After each dose of regular (immediate-release) carbidopa/levodopa, the standing BP will drop in susceptible people for about 3 to 4 hours (occasionally for only a couple of hours). This starts about 30 to 60 minutes after each dose. Subsequently, the BP returns to baseline. This pattern is important to appreciate so that the BP readings are done at appropriate times. The low BP levels are time-locked to individual carbidopa/levodopa doses.

In Chapter 6, we discussed the need to check the standing BP before starting carbidopa/levodopa. The systolic BP should be over 100 before initiating carbidopa/levodopa treatment. This provides a "cushion" based on the recognition that levodopa may lower the BP and that we want the BP readings over 90 (systolic).

If the initial BP is on the low side of normal (i.e., less than 120), the standing BP should be checked frequently after starting carbidopa/levodopa and after each dosage increment. The values should be recorded so that they can be shown to the clinician. If an increase in carbidopa/levodopa results in a drop in the systolic BP to 90 or less, the carbidopa/levodopa dosage should not be increased further. Before raising the doses, the low BP will need to be addressed, as discussed below.

Eating May Exacerbate Orthostatic Hypotension

Intake of food may contribute to orthostatic hypotension because blood flow to the gut increases when food is consumed. When a person is not eating, the blood vessels in the gastrointestinal system are reflexively constricted (when blood is not needed for digestion). The autonomic nervous system regulates this circulation; increased blood flow is required to meet the metabolic demands of digestion. With more blood going to the intestinal circulation during and after eating, people with orthostatic hypotension may experience an exacerbation of hypotensive symptoms. This phenomenon is called postprandial hypotension (*postprandial* means after eating; *hypotension* means low BP).

Factors Often Overlooked

Orthostatic hypotension is often not recognized because the tendency varies dramatically over the course of the day, influenced by specific factors. If the BP is measured when these factors are not operative, the BP will be normal. The principle factors are summarized as follows.

Linked to carbidopa/levodopa doses

Orthostatic hypotension is typically time-locked to carbidopa/levodopa doses. If the clinician checks the standing BP many hours after a dose of carbidopa/levodopa, the BP may be normal because the levodopa effect has dissipated.

Postprandial

Orthostatic hypotension is exacerbated by eating meals, especially large meals.

Morning exacerbation

After a night's sleep in bed, orthostatic hypotension is enhanced for several hours, often until lunchtime.

Other medications

When a water pill (diuretic) or pill for erectile dysfunction is taken, a transiently low BP may occur (see below).

Positional

Doctors and nurses conventionally check BP in the sitting position, thus missing a potential drop that may occur with standing.

These factors work against the detection of orthostatic hypotension. For example, a patient's BP may be normal, even when standing, if the clinic appointment is in the late afternoon, many hours after eating and carbidopa/levodopa administration.

When beginning routine BP measurements, it is good get in the habit of checking the BP after breakfast. For most people with orthostatic hypotension this will be the lowest reading of the day. That is because several exacerbating factors will be operative, including time of day (morning) and the fact that the reading is taken following a meal, and after carbidopa/levodopa (typically an hour before meals). Both the sitting and standing BP should be recorded so that these values can be provided to the clinician.

Beside routine checks of standing BP, it should also be measured when a person feels dizzy. It is important to check the BP in the position in which dizziness is present. As noted in the next section, dizziness may have different causes, and the clinician will be helped by such BP recordings.

What Else Might Cause Dizziness?

Dizziness is the term often communicated to the clinician when faintness is experienced. However, this word has other fundamentally different meanings. Dizziness also connotes imbalance, which most likely relates to parkinsonism rather than low BP. That form of dizziness is associated with a clear head.

Dizziness is also used for the sensation of vertigo. Episodic vertigo is common among older adults because of problems with the inner ear (vestibular system). Inner ear dizziness is experienced as spinning (vertigo) when it is severe, or head "wooziness" when the vestibular problem is mild. Vestibular vertigo is typically provoked by quick head movements or positions (e.g., turning over in bed or bending over).

A clue to vestibular dizziness is the position in which it occurs. Orthostatic hypotension should not be present when the person is lying and rarely when sitting. However, vestibular dizziness in the lying or sitting position is common. A sense of vertigo (spinning or illusory movement) is not a component of low BP and must be distinguished from it to avoid inappropriate treatment.

What Else Might Cause True Faintness?

The primary sensation of low BP is faintness or lightheadedness; if the BP is very low, fainting will occur. It is important to recognize, however, that there are other causes of true faintness. This is especially important if the faintness is experienced in discrete episodes, coming on suddenly in the absence of changes in body position. For example, sudden faintness while seated, which abates in a minute or two, is unlikely to be orthostatic hypotension. In that case, a cardiac cause and, specifically, a heart rhythm disturbance should be considered.

The heart typically beats regularly at a rate that efficiently allows filling of heart chambers, followed by heart muscle contractions to pump blood out to the major arteries. If the heart rate suddenly and inappropriately slows or stops, the BP will drop. Also, if the heart suddenly starts beating too rapidly, the rapid rate does not allow for filling between beats; this can also result in a drop in BP.

For such problems, assessment of the pulse should provide the clue to the cause. However, those clues are present only during the time of faintness; once the spell is over, the heart rate usually reverts to normal.

The pulse can be felt at the wrist (on the thumb side rather than the little finger side of the hand). To become good at counting the pulse, people can practice on themselves or a partner. Once familiar with how the pulse normally behaves, abnormal pulses become recognizable. An abnormal pulse during faintness will be faint and hard to feel, a characteristic that is important to note. The rate is also important; this is calculated by counting the number of beats per minute (e.g., count beats for 15 seconds and multiply by 4). A normal pulse rate is approximately

50 to 100 beats per minute and a little higher during exercise or excitement. Also, it is important to note if the pulse is regular, like a rhythmic drum beat (normal) or irregular, with varying pauses between beats.

The following are clues to a heart rhythm disturbance causing faintness: (1) sudden onset with brief symptoms lasting seconds to a few minutes; (2) occurrence when sitting or lying—that is, not orthostatic. Cardiac rhythm disturbances that cause episodic faintness need attention from the primary care doctor, internist, or cardiologist.

TREATMENT OF ORTHOSTATIC HYPOTENSION

If orthostatic hypotension is detected, there is a sequence of things to address, starting with the easiest. Treatment intensity depends on the standing BP. If the standing systolic BP is no higher than the low 80s, aggressive measures need to be taken, especially if the condition is symptomatic. With such low BP values, carbidopa/levodopa doses should not be raised until the orthostatic hypotension has been adequately treated. Doing first things first, scrutiny of the medication list is appropriate.

Many Medicines May Provoke Orthostatic Hypotension

Specific medications that tend to lower BP are too numerous to list here, so we will specify classes of drugs and examples. The patient's drug list should be reviewed with the primary care clinician, who can decide if potentially offending drugs can be safely reduced or eliminated.

Antihypertensives.

Many older adults are treated in mid-life for high BP (hypertension). If orthostatic hypotension later surfaces, such medications may need to be reduced or discontinued. Classes of antihypertensive drugs and common examples include the following.

Beta-blockers.

These drugs block adrenalin-like substances. They are also used for rapid heart rates, certain other cardiac conditions, migraines, and essential tremor. Common beta-blockers include atenolol (Tenormin), metoprolol (Lopressor, Toprol), propranolol (Inderal), nadolol (Corgard), timolol (Blocadren), and pindolol (Visken).

Calcium-channel blockers.

This medication class is also used for other conditions besides high BP, including migraine and certain heart conditions. Commonly prescribed calcium-channel blockers include verapamil (Calan, Isoptin, Verelan), diltiazem (Cardizem, Tiazac, Dilacor), nifedipine (Adalat, Procardia), amlodipine (Norvasc), isradipine (DynaCirc), felodipine (Plendil), and nicardipine (Cardene).

ACE-inhibitors.

These drugs block angiotensin converting enzyme (ACE), which is an enzyme in the kidney's system for maintaining BP. This class of drug is also used in treatment of diabetes mellitus and heart disease. ACE inhibitors include lisinopril (Prinivil, Zestril), enalapril (Vasotec), quinapril (Accupril), benazepril (Lotensin), ramipril (Altace), and captopril (Capoten).

Angiotensin II-receptor blockers.

Angiotensin II is a hormone that constricts blood vessels and elevates BP; blocking it will lower BP. Drugs from this class include valsartan (Diovan), losartan (Cozaar), irbesartan (Avapro), candesartan (Atacand), and telmisartan (Micardis).

Diuretics (water pills).

Diuretics are often part of antihypertensive (high BP) treatment. They also are the primary medication to treat swelling (edema) and are used for congestive heart failure. If the indication for the diuretic is not serious it may be possible to discontinue it. For example, leg swelling could alternatively be treated by elevating the legs and wearing support hose. Commonly prescribed diuretics include hydrochlorothiazide (HCTZ), furosemide (Lasix), triamterene (usually combined with HCTZ; Dyazide), chlorthalidone, indapamide (Lozol), amiloride (Midamor), torsemide (Demadex), and spironolactone (Aldactone).

Prostate hypertrophy pills: alpha-blockers.

There are two classes of medicines for reducing an enlarged prostate (impeding urine flow). Only one of these is problematic for people with orthostatic hypotension: alpha-blockers. The most commonly prescribed drug in this class is tamsulosin (Flomax). Others include doxazosin (Cardura), terazosin (Hytrin), silodosin (Rapaflo) and alfuzosin (Uroxatral).

Specific heart drugs.

If the patient has a serious cardiac disorder, elimination of certain heart drugs may not be advisable. This decision requires review and approval by the cardiologist or primary care physician. The main offenders overlap with the antihypertensive and diuretic drugs listed above. A common drug from this group that potently lowers BP is carvedilol (Coreg). Typically it is prescribed for serious heart disease and usually cannot be discontinued.

Male erectile dysfunction drugs.

If symptomatic orthostatic hypotension is diagnosed, it would be wise to avoid sildenafil (Viagra), vardenafil (Levitra), or tadalafil (Cialis) as they tend to lower BP.

Antidepressants.

The older drugs from this class, tricyclic antidepressants, have the potential for exacerbating orthostatic hypotension, although this effect is usually modest. They are also used for other purposes such as treating migraine, chronic pain, or sleep. The commonly prescribed drugs from the tricyclic class include nortriptyline (Pamelor), amitriptyline (Elavil), protriptyline (Vivactil), imipramine (Tofranil), and desipramine (Norpramin). Other antidepressants with potential for exacerbating orthostatic hypotension include doxepin (Sinequan) and mirtazapine (Remeron). Trazodone may also do this, but it is not a major offender when used in low doses for sleep, which accounts for most prescriptions.

The medications listed above do not comprise an exhaustive list of those with potential for provoking orthostatic hypotension, but they do provide a starting point when reviewing the medication list with the clinician in the event of orthostatic hypotension.

Low BP While Sitting

If a low BP is present while the person is sitting as well as standing the clinician should address this, as the blood volume may be deficient. For example, such low BP may reflect anemia. It may also be present with fluid loss due to vomiting or diarrhea.

Treatment of Orthostatic Hypotension Without Adding Drugs

The primary goal for treating orthostatic hypotension is to avoid faints, near-faints, or light-headedness when the person is up and about. Again, the upright systolic BP should be maintained above 90. When orthostatic hypotension becomes apparent, it is important to work with the clinician in managing this, starting with recording the BP values.

The standing BP should be checked routinely after breakfast, occasionally at other times, and whenever dizziness is experienced. The sitting BP should occasionally be measured as well.

Once it appears that orthostatic hypotension needs to be treated, there are several simple things that are initially appropriate to do:

1. Review the medication list with the clinician and eliminate contributors to low BPs, if possible (see above).
2. Increase fluid intake (e.g., 6 to 8 tall glasses daily of some fluid).
3. Increase salt intake (many older adults restrict salt intake).

Note that the reduction of BP due to carbidopa/levodopa is dose-related. In other words, the higher the dose, the lower the BP. If a certain dosage of levodopa is necessary to maintain ambulation, then a lower one may not be an option. However, if higher doses add little benefit, then lowering the carbidopa/levodopa dosage may help. Recall that the BP reduction is linked to each dose, not the total daily dose.

Compressive hose.

Wearing of compressive hose (thigh- or waist-high) can help prevent blood from pooling in the lower half of the body. People with orthostatic hypotension have lost reflexive constriction of blood vessels in their legs. Normally, the act of standing triggers blood vessel constriction via the autonomic nervous system. Without this, gravity pulls the blood to the feet. In orthostatic hypotension, where this reflex is lost, vessels in the legs dilate, blood pools there, and the BP drops.

If the blood vessels no longer constrict with standing, a simple approach is to keep them constricted by means of outside pressure. In other words, a uniform compression of the legs counters this problem. Compressive hose may be purchased to provide this outside pressure. They are expensive and must be a properly fitted, but they do the job. Note, however, that the entirety of the lower limbs must be externally constricted for this to work; knee-high compressive hose are ineffective (the type of hose often routinely used among hospitalized patients). The hose must be a snug fit through the thighs and ideally waist-high. Tight bands (e.g., rubber bands) must be avoided since localized constriction of blood flow in the veins can cause clots, which are dangerous (deep vein thromboses).

The clinician can provide a prescription for compressive hose, specifying either thigh-high or waist-high hose. The latter are similar to snug-fitting panty hose. Medical supply stores and large pharmacies are good sources. The waist-high hose are preferable but may be hard to quickly remove for people with urinary urgency. The prescription will need to specify the extent of compression, which may be 15–20 mmHg, 20–30 mmHg, or 30–40 mmHg (note that millimeters of mercury is the unit of measurement, as for BP). Often the 20–30 mmHg size is tried first. Again, these hose need to be fitted, matched to leg size.

The hose are put on each morning, preferably before getting out of bed, and taken off at night. Putting them on and taking them off can be difficult and sometimes requires a helper (care partner). Using the old-fashioned dishwashing gloves with good finger traction is often helpful. The major limitation of these hose is the hassle factor. They can also be uncomfortable to wear in warm climates. The hose contain elastic and require gentle washing (not with hot water), using mild detergents to avoid degrading the elastic.

Abdominal binder.

Better control of orthostatic hypotension can be obtained by adding an abdominal binder, available via a medical supply store or large pharmacy. The special benefit of this binder is that it helps counter the tendency of the gastrointestinal blood vessels to open (dilate) during meal digestion, which may cause postprandial hypotension. The binder resembles the girdles women wore that were popular in prior generations. The binder is tightened with Velcro straps. Some people with orthostatic hypotension who cannot tolerate the compressive hose can still benefit from wearing the abdominal binder. If it is prescribed, purchase of the binder, as well as the hose, may be reimbursed.

Drugs to Raise Blood Pressure

Fludrocortisone (Florinef).

Fludrocortisone prevents the kidneys from eliminating ingested salt (sodium) into the urine. It is typically started at a dose of 0.1 mg once daily, then twice daily if necessary. It takes at least a week to be effective. It may be raised up to 0.2 mg twice daily. It is unclear if higher doses provide incremental benefit. Fludrocortisone has only a modest ability to elevate BP and also does this around the clock, with the potential for raising the BP when the person is in bed at night. Fludrocortisone requires liberal salt intake for it to work. If it is consistently used, the primary care provider should occasionally check the blood levels of sodium and potassium.

Extra carbidopa (Lodosyn).

In Chapter 6, we discussed taking extra carbidopa to prevent nausea. Sometimes that same strategy works for treatment of orthostatic hypotension. It is harmless to try. Thus, two plain carbidopa (Lodosyn) 25 mg tablets can be taken with each dose of carbidopa/levodopa. This is more likely to work when the carbidopa/levodopa dose provoking orthostatic hypotension is two tablets or less.

Midodrine (ProAmatine).

If the above strategies prove insufficient and faintness remains problematic, adding midodrine is an appropriate next step. To be used effectively, knowledge of how this drug works is required.

In DLB and PDD, low BP levels are usually driven by each dose of carbidopa/levodopa. Eliminating carbidopa/levodopa would theoretically solve the problem but, in return, compromise movement. When low BP levels are time-locked to each dose of carbidopa/levodopa, a simple solution is to add the BP-elevating drug, midodrine, which has about the same response duration as carbidopa/levodopa. As discussed earlier, carbidopa/levodopa lowers the standing BP for about 3 to 4 hours. Midodrine has approximately the same duration of action but the opposite effect on BP; it raises the BP for about 4 hours after each dose. Hence, midodrine taken with each dose of carbidopa/levodopa will tend to counter the BP-lowering effect of levodopa—they offset one another.

Conventionally, midodrine is started with a single 2.5 mg tablet taken with each daytime dose of carbidopa/levodopa. The standing BP readings recorded 1 to 2 hours later will indicate if the dosage is adequate. If insufficient, midodrine is then raised to 5 mg each dose. Parenthetically, 2.5 mg is too low for the needs of most patients. Thus, if the BP is markedly low, it may be appropriate to start with 5 mg midodrine for each dose. Dose escalation is guided by the BP. If the BP is still too low (less than 90 systolic, standing), then the midodrine dose is raised from 5 to 7.5 mg, which is usually adequate. Occasionally, patients need higher doses, going to 10 mg, and ultimately up to 15 mg each dose. Midodrine should not be taken before bedtime or during the night, as it can raise the BP to excessive levels when a person is lying down.

Remember that midodrine raises the BP for about 4 hours. If carbidopa/levodopa is not being used, then midodrine is typically taken every 4 hours during the waking day (but not within 4 hours of bedtime). Sometimes the printed midodrine instructions stipulate taking it three times daily; however, that will not cover the waking day unless a person spends 12 hours in bed each day.

Note that if carbidopa/levodopa is taken every 2 hours, it would then make sense to take the midodrine with every other dose, since it lasts 4 hours. Midodrine does not have many side effects; some people experience tingling or similar skin sensations.

Pyridostigmine (Mestinon).

A disorder called myasthenia gravis is routinely treated with pyridostigmine, which enhances the activity of a neurotransmitter called acetylcholine. Pyridostigmine does not get into the brain but has widespread effects in the body. One important effect is countering the tendency toward orthostatic hypotension. Pyridostigmine does not raise the BP when a person is sitting or lying, only in the standing position. Like midodrine, it does this for about 4 hours. It usually is added to midodrine, but occasionally it is used alone. The effects on BP are not as prominent as with midodrine. Certainly one advantage, however, is that it does not contribute to supine hypertension (high BP when lying down). Pyridostigmine is typically started at a dose of 30 mg, either with each dose of midodrine and carbidopa/levodopa, or every 4 hours. If 30 mg (one-half of a 60 mg tablet) is insufficient it can be raised to 60 mg, then 90 mg. Usually individual doses are not raised past 90 to 120 mg. There is also a sustained-release tablet, but this is not routinely used in this setting because the effect is not predictable and does not last all day.

Side effects from pyridostigmine include an increase in gastrointestinal activity, including loose stools. It may also increase salivation and sweating, although these are rarely consequential.

What to Do If the BP Is Too High When Lying Down?

When trying to raise the standing BP, the BP when lying in bed may become too high. It is difficult to achieve perfect control, and often a slightly high BP in bed may have to be accepted.

If the lying BP is over 160 systolic or 100 diastolic (the bottom BP number), then six-inch blocks can be placed under the head of the bed to will allow gravity to lower the BP (pulling blood to the feet). This is the same strategy used for heartburn (gastric reflux).

Lying BP values that remain quite high, such as over 200 systolic or 110 diastolic, should be discussed with the clinician. If this happens only occasionally it may be acceptable; however, if it is a frequent occurrence it may require treatment. Treatment may include reducing one of the BP-elevating medications listed above. Rarely, a short-acting BP-lowering drug, such as hydralazine (5 to 10 mg), may be given before bedtime. However, this can cause too low a BP if the person gets up to go to the bathroom at night, and one could faint on the way there. This can be a difficult treatment situation and mildly elevated BP levels may need to be accepted.

14

Bladder Problems

Urinary problems occur with normal aging. In women they often relate to the changes in female anatomy due to the delivering of babies. With superimposed age-related changes in soft tissues, laxity may result in incontinence (loss of urinary control), especially with coughing, laughing, or straining. In men the opposite symptom tends to occur: urinary hesitancy (inability to evacuate the bladder). This is due to constriction of the bladder outlet by an enlarging prostate; the prostate normally surrounds the urethra, through which urine passes.

DLB and PDD are often associated with additional bladder problems. Recall that the autonomic nervous system regulates bladder function and that this system tends to malfunction in Lewy disorders. Hence, reduced bladder control is frequent among those with DLB, PDD, and Parkinson's disease. This condition is termed neurogenic bladder, which implies that the autonomic nervous system control of bladder reflexes is not working properly. This may manifest as urgency with incontinence or hesitancy. Neurogenic bladder problems require different strategies than those used for treating the simple age-related problems that develop in mid-life and beyond. Moreover, there are certain caveats to treatment once a neurogenic bladder is recognized.

BACKGROUND ON THE BLADDER

The bladder is simply a reservoir that holds urine. It is located in the lower pelvis and is distant from the kidneys. The kidneys essentially filter the circulating blood and make the urine. The urine flows down from the kidneys into the bladder, as shown in Figure 14.1. Normally, as the bladder slowly fills with urine, a reflex is triggered when it is nearly full. This results in conscious awareness of the need to urinate, plus it primes the reflexive tendency of the bladder to contract in order to expel the urinary contents.

The bladder is able to contract because of muscles in the bladder walls. Normally, nerves activate these muscles at the appropriate time, which forcefully squeeze the bladder, expelling the urine. Nerve sensors in the bladder wall are activated by bladder filling and transmit this information to the central nervous system, ramping up bladder wall muscle activity. When this mechanism works properly, urination occurs with no conscious effort, apart from recognizing the need to walk to the bathroom and allowing this to occur.

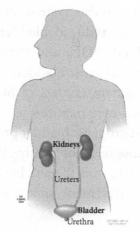

Figure 14.1 The urinary system, from kidneys to bladder, with urine expelled via the urethra.

Normal aging in woman impairs the ability of the bladder outlet to prevent leakage of urine. In men, overgrowth of the prostate (prostatism) squeezes the bladder outlet (urethra), preventing urine from being expelled. Since the prostate surrounds the urethra, any enlargement will indeed tend to squeeze the outlet shut.

If the bladder is unable to expel urine, the retained urine can become a nidus for infection. This could be due to constriction of the urethra, weak bladder wall muscles, or stretching of the bladder walls. It may also be caused by a neurogenic bladder. Urinary tract infections (UTIs) are sometimes the first signal of bladder problems. The symptoms of infection may include urinary urgency, painful urination (dysuria), malodorous urine, or further impairment of urinary control.

INVOLVE A UROLOGIST

A neurogenic bladder due to Lewy processes may cause urinary hesitancy, incontinence, or both. Hence, it can be mistaken for male prostatism or female anatomy–related incontinence. Sometimes there is more than one problem causing the urinary symptoms. It is difficult to sort this out without testing. The appropriate tests are done by urologists. It is important to inform the urologist that DLB or PDD is present so that they can be aware of the potential for a neurogenic bladder.

If a urinary infection has been excluded by urinalysis, a urologist will often proceed with two procedures. One is cystoscopy, in which an endoscope is inserted through the urethra into the bladder. This allows the urologist to examine the inside walls of the bladder and make certain that there are no mechanical impediments to flow, and to exclude cancers. The other test is called urodynamics, which is used to analyze bladder reflexes. These procedures do not need to be done repeatedly but usually just once to document the reason for the urinary symptoms.

An additional study typically performed to further assess a hesitant bladder is catheterization after the urine is voluntarily voided. What is left over is termed the residual urine. In general, residual urine should be kept to a minimum, as old urine in the bladder can be a source of infection.

TREATMENT

Simple Things

If the patient is taking a water pill (diuretic), this will generate additional urine. In some people such a drug may not be necessary; this can be discussed with the clinician. Coffee, tea, and caffeinated soda pop tend to have a diuretic effect; intake of these should be considered as appropriate. Urinary tract infections need to be treated, as discussed later in this chapter.

If the person is frequently urinating at night (nocturia), fluid intake after supper should be minimized. If urgency or incontinence is present, fluid intake should be reduced before going out. Pads or disposable padded underwear are very useful for dealing with incontinence.

Drugs for Urinary Urgency and Urge Incontinence

A bladder that is too quick to contract is termed a hyperactive bladder. This is the basis for urinary urgency. Medications used to dampen this tendency block a neurotransmitter in the bladder wall, acetylcholine (anticholinergics). Unfortunately, most of these anticholinergic medications can pass into the brain and block acetylcholine receptors in memory centers; drugs with such potential to impair memory were listed in Table 12.1. These drugs may also contribute to hallucinations (Chapter 10). Hence, the anticholinergic drugs shown in Table 12.1 should be avoided in the setting of DLB or PDD. The one anticholinergic medication that spares memory is trospium (Sanctura). Trospium has a molecular configuration that will not allow it to cross the blood–brain barrier and thus works only outside the brain. However, like the other anticholinergic drugs, a variety of other side effects may be provoked, including dry mouth and eyes, constipation, slowed stomach emptying, and visual blurring. Trospium is typically administered as a 20 mg tablet twice daily. If urinary urgency is only problematic at night it can be taken as a single bedtime dose (or morning dose for urgency primarily during the day time). A long-acting form taken once daily is also available (60 mg).

Urinary tract infections will often be associated with urgency or urge incontinence. All infections should be addressed before starting drugs to slow the urinary stream. An infection may need to be revisited if new urinary symptoms arise.

Treatment of Urinary Hesitancy

A neurogenic bladder that does not expel the urine (hypoactive bladder) can be difficult to treat. Pills are not very effective for this if there is no obstruction (e.g., not due to prostate enlargement). Rarely, the bladder outlet muscle is too contracted, and this can be treated with injection of botulinum toxin. However, those with a hypoactive neurogenic bladder usually have "lazy" muscles in the bladder wall that poorly contract. In that case, a sterile tube (catheter) can be inserted into the bladder to remove the urine. Catheterization, however, can introduce bacteria and incite a urinary infection. Catheterization is typically managed by urologists if it is necessary to do this chronically or on a frequent basis.

Urologists continue to work on surgical interventions for loss of bladder control, so better treatments may be on the horizon.

Urinary Hesitancy: Treatment to Avoid

Normal, middle-aged men with an enlarged prostate often have difficulty passing urine. Surgical removal of prostate tissue to relieve the compression is typically curative. This procedure is termed transurethral resection of prostate (TURP). Men with DLB or PDD and urinary hesitancy due to a neurogenic bladder are poor candidates for a TURP; it can convert urinary hesitancy into urinary incontinence. Urinary incontinence is typically less well tolerated than a mildly slowed urinary stream.

TREATMENT OF URINARY TRACT INFECTIONS (UTIs)

We have already emphasized the importance of treating UTIs. Unfortunately, among those with poorly contracting hypoactive bladders the residual urine easily grows bacteria. Trying to completely and consistently eradicate the bacteria is sometimes a losing battle. Moreover, ongoing antibiotic treatment may select out resistant bacteria, making subsequent antibiotic treatment difficult. Clinicians are well aware of this dilemma and try to keep the urine as sterile as possible without generating a new generation of hard-to-treat organisms. This is complicated territory, and for such problems, close alliance with the clinician is important. There are many types of antibiotics and strategies for minimizing urine bacterial counts. A good clinician will recognize the limitations, side effects, and potential to cause new and more complicated problems with these drugs.

How to Diagnose a Urinary Tract Infection

Symptoms typically signal the need to consider a UTI and may include pain on urination, urinary urgency, bladder discomfort (lower pelvis), or very malodorous or cloudy urine.

The test for a UTI includes a urinalysis, at the very minimum. If it shows many white cells and bacteria, this is suggestive of a UTI. White cells are the body's defense against bacteria; their presence indicates that an infection is being fought by the immune system. Beyond the urinalysis, a urine culture is often appropriate; it confirms the presence of bacteria and the specific type.

Usually, there is one predominant strain of bacteria causing the infection. Once identified, the laboratory can then test the culture-grown bacteria against different antibiotics. The results will help the clinician identify which antibiotic(s) will kill the bacteria isolated from that urine sample.

Urinary Tract Infections May Trigger Neurologic Decline

In the context of DLB and PDD, urinary infections (like any infection) can occasionally cause an episode of confusion or neurologic deterioration. Even if there are no clear urinary symptoms, a urinalysis should be included in the evaluation of recent-onset neurologic decline, as discussed in Chapter 12. Note that UTIs may be present without symptoms.

Urinary Drugs that May Need to Be Stopped

We have already discussed anticholinergic drugs for hyperactive bladder (urinary urgency) that can worsen memory and occasionally provoke hallucinations. As detailed above, if a drug for hyperactive bladder is advised, trospium should be the choice in the setting of DLB or PDD.

Men with an enlarged prostate may have trouble urinating. Urologists typically prescribe alpha-blockers for this problem, which block adrenalin-like substances. These drugs are also notorious for lowering the blood pressure and include tamsulosin (Flomax), doxazosin (Cardura), terazosin (Hytrin), silodosin (Rapaflo) and alfuzosin (Uroxatral). If orthostatic hypotension is a problem, then these should not be used.

Another class of drugs for enlarged prostate, the 5-alpha-reductase inhibitors, do not lower blood pressure. These include finasteride (Proscan) and dutasteride (Avodart) and may be used in the setting of DLB or PDD. However, these take many months to work, so urologists often prescribe an alpha-blocker at the same time for more immediate results.

15

Bowels and Constipation

Constipation is common among older adults, in general. However, it is very common among people with Lewy body disorders, and the reason is dysautonomia. Lewy body disorders tend to impair control of gut motility by the autonomic nervous system. At the stomach level, bloating may develop when the stomach fails to empty into the upper small intestine. At the other end, constipation is the consequence of Lewy processes affecting motility in the colon. Colon motility (peristalsis) is what moves the remnants of digested food (stool) to the rectum for expulsion. These regions are shown in Figure 15.1.

ANTICHOLINERGIC DRUGS EXACERBATE CONSTIPATION

Drugs that block the neurotransmitter acetylcholine are notorious for worsening constipation; these include medications used to treat urinary urgency (overactive bladder). All of the anticholinergic drugs for bladder overactivity that were listed in Table 12.1 cause constipation, as does another bladder drug, trospium (Sanctura). The tricyclic drugs for depression shown in Table 12.1 have variable anticholinergic properties and also

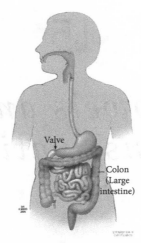

Figure 15.1 Gastrointestinal system from mouth to esophagus, to stomach, then to small intestine and, finally, colon.

tend to be constipating. One needs to balance benefits against the side effect of constipation if considering these medications.

IS ALL CONSTIPATION THIS SIMPLE?

In the setting of DLB or PDD, constipation is typically due to autonomic nervous system dysfunction, often exacerbated by medication side effects. However, there are exceptions and the primary care clinician or internist should consider whether colonoscopy is appropriate. This procedure involves inserting a scope into the anus and then advancing the instrument to visualize the entire colon. In this way hidden colon cancers are detected before they become deadly.

TREATMENT OF CONSTIPATION

Routine Measures

It is common knowledge that several natural remedies help prevent constipation: fruits, vegetables, fluids, and fiber. Individuals with constipation should make sure that their diet includes adequate fruits, which make a good snack. Meals should include vegetables, such as green beans, peas, and squash; catsup and potatoes do not count as vegetables. Intake of six to eight tall glasses of water, juice, or other fluids may help maintain moisture in the stool, making it easier to pass. Finally, fiber needs to be included in the diet in order to give the stool bulk. These strategies are often insufficient for persons with Lewy disorders, and additional measures are often necessary.

Goals

It is not imperative that we have a bowel movement every day, but a reasonable goal is to have a good bowel movement every 2 to 3 days. If many days elapse between bowel movements, there is the increasing likelihood that the stool in the colon will become dry (desiccated) and more difficult to evacuate. This problem is discussed further below, in the section "Chronic Constipation with Impaction."

Constipation Not Responding to Simple Measures

As mentioned earlier, diet and fluids are often inadequate means of addressing constipation in those with DLB and PDD and thus a laxative is often necessary. For regular use, certain laxatives are better than others, and clinicians generally recommend laxatives that work by osmotic factors. These contain unabsorbable particles that draw water into the gut (by osmosis). The alternative, stimulant laxatives, work by directly causing the gut to contract. Stimulant laxatives may work well for a short time but may become less effective if used regularly and can cause dependence.

Perhaps the most commonly recommended osmotic laxatives are those containing polyethylene glycol. This type comes as a powder that is dissolved in a solution (e.g., water, juice) and drank. It is sold as over-the-counter MiraLax or PEG 3350. This is a reasonable choice, following the directions on the package.

Another laxative that can be used for chronic constipation is lubiprostone (Amitiza), which also appears helpful for treating constipation in those with Lewy disorders; it requires a prescription.

Generally, it is appropriate to see if the simple diet and fluid measures enable a bowel movement. However, if 2 days elapse without success, then a laxative may be considered. With an osmotic laxative, this can be done on a regular, ongoing basis.

If a week or so has elapsed without a bowel movement, stool in the colon may become hard and not be very moveable. In that case, a laxative may provoke abdominal cramping. In other words, the colon may be trying to contract, but is obstructed by hard, impacted stool that will not move. Other strategies are then necessary, as discussed in the next section. If this problem develops it should be discussed with the clinician. Rarely, other problems in the colon may produce the same symptoms, including obstructing tumors.

Chronic Constipation with Impaction

If the stool in the colon does not move for many days it may dry out (become desiccated) and hard to move. The colon is a long tube, and old stool can back up and prevent passage (impaction). If this happens, laxatives may not work and simply cause cramps. If impacted stool is the problem, there will be no formed bowel movements but instead watery diarrhea may occur. In fact, watery diarrhea may leak without control (incontinence). This may initially seem confusing: severe constipation, yet diarrhea. The likelihood is that impacted stool prevents passage of formed feces, whereas watery stool can leak around it. This may be a sign of impaction.

The approach to impacted stool is to clean it out, whether associated with watery leakage or not. This often requires a high-volume enema; note that Fleet-brand and similar enemas on pharmacy shelves are typically low volume (7.8 ounces; 230 mL). These are appropriate for the milder problems of the general public, when the nonmoving stool is at the very end of the colon in the rectum. For that problem not much fluid is necessary. For people with refractory constipation who have gone many days without a bowel movement, the impacted stool may well be much further back in the colon and require much larger volumes of fluid to reach it. The intent is to soak and lubricate the hard, impacted stool that is higher up in the colon, enabling it to move out.

The typical volume of fluid used for this type of enema is approximately 1 liter (around a quart). The most convenient fluid to use is tap water that is slightly warm (i.e., similar temperature to the body). An enema kit for this purpose can be purchased at a drug store. This process typically requires someone to administer the enema. It is done with the constipated person lying on his or her side close to the toilet. The enema tube is lubricated and inserted into the rectum (via the anus). The other end is connected to a fluid container holding the tap water. The fluid in the container is allowed to flow, using gravity as the force. In other words, raising the fluid reservoir produces the pressure needed to push the water into the rectum and colon. The higher the receptacle, the higher the pressure. As the fluid fills the colon, an urge to have a bowel movement typically occurs; this is the signal to get up and sit on the toilet. This process may need to be repeated. This can be a messy job, so one needs to be prepared.

Once the colon is cleaned out, the simpler strategy of diet and fluids, plus intermittent laxatives, should then allow bowel movements on subsequent days. If the bowels can be kept moving, impaction should be avoided.

OTHER SLEEP PROBLEMS

Previously we discussed how insomnia is common in DLB and PDD, emphasizing that it can often be effectively treated with appropriate dosing and timing of carbidopa/levodopa. Other sleep problems may also affect people with DLB and PDD. These are treatable and will be addressed in the next two chapters.

16

Daytime Drowsiness

Drowsiness is common in those with DLB and PDD, and can interfere with thinking and memory, as well as quality of life. There are a variety of potential reasons for this, many treatable.

WHEN IS DAYTIME DROWSINESS PATHOLOGIC?

Getting a little sleepy during a boring task or napping after lunch on the weekend is not a sign of a medical problem. However, daytime drowsiness should draw attention in certain circumstances:

1. More than one nap most days, or near-daily naps that span 2 to 3 hours
2. Falling asleep during conversations or eating
3. Frequently falling asleep during reading, watching TV, doing computer work or other vigilant tasks
4. Returning to sleep after breakfast

These are signs that could indicate that nighttime sleep was not adequate (nonrestorative) but could have other explanations.

CAUSES

Daytime drowsiness has limited causes:

1. Insomnia at bedtime
2. Awakening during the night

3. Insufficient time spent in bed at night
4. Poor quality sleep at night (despite adequate time in bed)
5. Daytime medications inducing drowsiness
6. A primary sleep disorder directly causing drowsiness (which may be DLB or PDD related).

We will explore each of these possible causes and how they might be diagnosed and treated. If a person with DLB or PDD is excessively drowsy, at least one of these could be the problem.

INSOMNIA CAUSING DAYTIME DROWSINESS

Inability to get to sleep at bedtime can translate into sleepiness during the daytime. Many people with DLB or PDD who experience insomnia benefit from nighttime carbidopa/levodopa doses. The benefits of carbidopa/levodopa dosing at bedtime for Lewy-related insomnia were addressed in Chapter 9. Various other factors, however, may contribute to insomnia.

Drugs Keeping You Awake

Sometimes medications taken in the evening are alerting. Such drugs include duloxetine (Cymbalta) or venlafaxine (Effexor), used for depression and often dosed twice daily. Elimination of all but the morning dose may allow sleep in such cases. Other drugs for depression from the Prozac class (SSRIs; see the list in Chapter 18) may also cause insomnia if taken at bedtime. A simple strategy is to simply switch to morning dosing on a trial basis. The tricyclic antidepressants, such as nortriptyline, amitriptyline, or protriptyline, should not cause insomnia; they may induce sleep.

Occasionally, sleepy people are prescribed stimulants with long-acting properties, such as extended-release methylphenidate (Concerta), modafinil (Provigil), or armodafinil (Nuvigil).

The alerting effects may extend to bedtime. Evening consumption of caffeinated beverages may have the same effect.

Restless Legs Syndrome

Restless legs syndrome (RLS) is fairly common among adults and may be the reason for insomnia. It manifests as a creepy-crawly, tingling, or similar sensation in the legs beginning in the evening or at bedtime. It is relieved by movement and sometimes requires the sleeper to get up and walk around for relief.

RLS is primarily treated with medications that promote dopamine transmission in the brain, including carbidopa/levodopa or dopamine agonists. The dopamine agonists pramipexole (Mirapex), ropinirole (Requip), and rotigotine (Neupro) are the usual medications selected for RLS treatment in the general population. Carbidopa/levodopa is also effective but is a second-line choice for reasons discussed below. As discussed in Chapter 5, dopamine agonists are substantially more likely to induce hallucinations than carbidopa/levodopa. Hence, they are usually not the first choice for treatment of RLS in people with DLB or PDD. If someone with DLB or PDD is already taking one of these dopamine agonists for RLS with good success, the drug may be continued (but switched if hallucinations surface).

Carbidopa/levodopa works well for RLS in the general population, but after several weeks the restless legs symptoms may surface earlier in the day, requiring another carbidopa/levodopa dose. Eventually, levodopa dosing may be necessary several times during the day. This situation is termed rebound or augmentation. This is not a major issue for people with Parkinson's disease, DLB, or PDD who already take several doses of carbidopa/levodopa for their parkinsonian symptoms. For those taking three carbidopa/levodopa doses during the waking day and who also have nighttime restless legs, a carbidopa/levodopa dose an hour before bedtime is a reasonable treatment strategy. It may be repeated during the night, if necessary.

SLEEP AIDS

Sleep Hygiene

Falling asleep requires a proper state of mind and environment. General strategies include the following:

1. Avoid stressful activities in the evening. Although exercise typically promotes good sleep, some people find it energizing before bedtime. Similarly, avoid starting exciting or stimulating activities before bed. Make the evening a time to wind down from the day's activities.

2. Do not nap in the evening and do not take long naps during the day. Sleeping during the daytime tends to reset the biological clock so that you are not tired at night. To reset it, do not sleep during the day (although a short, 30- to 60-minute nap after lunch is acceptable). If tending to nap after supper, avoid sedentary activities that promote this.

3. Establish a regular sleep routine, generally retiring around the same time each night.

4. Set aside the bedroom for sleep and do not use it for other activities. Sleep in a dark room. Do not leave the TV on. The intent is to associate a dark, quiet bedroom with sleep.

5. Choose a bedroom temperature conducive to sleep; often this is a slightly cooler room.

6. Do exercise; strenuous exercise earlier in the day promotes good sleep at night.

7. Do not overeat right before bed. An overfilled stomach may provoke heartburn (gastric reflux).

8. Avoid clock-watching during the night.

Finally, do not use alcoholic beverages as a sleep aid. Although they promote getting to sleep, the effect is transient and often associated with awakening during the night.

Over-the-Counter Sleep Aids

Again, it is worth reiterating that a full dose of carbidopa/levodopa may be the best sleep aid in DLB and PDD (see Chapter 9). However, that may not solve insomnia for everyone. If unable to get to sleep and the above strategies have proven insufficient, a sleep aid may be tried. There are two over-the-counter sleep aids that may be helpful, melatonin and diphenhydramine.

Melatonin is a natural hormone made by the pineal gland (located in the central region of the brain). It is important for maintenance of the body's day–night cycle, and it helps promote sleep. It is widely available over the counter at drug stores and grocery store drug counters. It typically is administered as a 1 mg or 3 mg tablet/capsule, taken at least an hour before bedtime. It can be raised by 1 mg to 3 mg increments up to 6 mg as a single dose; occasionally, doses as high as 12 mg are tried, although it is unclear if such higher doses have any advantage. Melatonin should not cause nocturnal confusion or imbalance (a concern with some sedating sleep aids).

Diphenhydramine directly induces drowsiness. It was primarily used years ago as an antihistamine for allergic symptoms. Antihistamines that pass into the brain induce drowsiness. Because diphenhydramine is so sedating, it no longer is used to treat allergies, being supplanted by new antihistamines that do not get into the brain. Diphenhydramine is available over the counter in a variety of brand-name products, including Benadryl. It is administered before bedtime in doses of 25 to 50 mg. It is found in combination drugs advocated for sleep, such as Tylenol PM (500 mg acetaminophen and 25 mg diphenhydramine) and Advil PM (200 mg ibuprofen and 38 mg diphenhydramine). Diphenhydramine occasionally causes confusion during the night. It is typically administered 30 to 60 minutes before bedtime.

Short-Acting Prescription Sleep Aids

There has been a proliferation of prescription drugs that induce sleep but without persistent drowsiness, thus usually avoiding grogginess the next morning. Occasionally, with such sleep aids, awakening may occur a few hours into the night. In that case, a second dose is sometimes used. Drugs in this class include zolpidem (Ambien), zaleplon (Sonata), and eszopiclone (Lunesta). These and related drugs run the risk of nighttime confusion or fall risk on the way to the bathroom. They may also lead to dependence. Uncommonly, there may be carryover effects in the morning.

Sedating Antidepressant Drugs Used in Low Doses as Sleep Aids

Trazodone is the prototypic antidepressant medication used as a sleep aid. It is typically started at a dose of 50 mg an hour or so before bedtime. The dose can be raised to 100 mg and sometimes slightly higher as necessary. This has longer-lasting effects that sometimes promote a full night's sleep. However, nighttime sedation can be problematic if arising to go to the bathroom.

Other medications from this class that are similarly used in low doses for sleep include amitriptyline, nortriptyline, and doxepin (each administered in doses of 10 to 50 mg at bedtime). These latter three drugs do have anticholinergic properties, albeit mild in such low doses. Anticholinergics can impair memory and bowel motility.

Finally, mirtazapine (Remeron), which is an antidepressant drug from a different class, is also used for sleep (15 mg).

Anti-Hallucination Drug Used as Sleep Aid

Quetiapine (Seroquel) was discussed in Chapter 10 as a medication to counter hallucinations and delusions (antipsychotic). That is the proper indication for this medication. However, an added benefit is its sedating property, which often persists throughout the night. Most clinicians would not prescribe it solely as a sleep aid.

AWAKENING DURING THE NIGHT

Frequent awakening is problematic if it is difficult to return to sleep. Moreover, this often disrupts the sleep of spouses, partners and caregivers. There are a variety of reasons for frequent awakening, each with specific treatment strategies.

Awakening from Dopamine Deficiency

As discussed in Chapter 4, those with DLB and PDD have deficiencies of brain dopamine. The conventional three-times daily carbidopa/levodopa dosing schedule may not adequately replenish brain dopamine at night. Those with short-duration levodopa responses may awaken due to the levodopa effect wearing off (discussed in Chapter 9). For those with this problem, a variety of symptoms surface that tend to awaken individuals and prevent them from returning to sleep. This includes a feeling of inner restlessness (similar but not identical to restless legs syndrome) or an inability to get comfortable or to turn in bed.

As discussed earlier, a full dose of carbidopa/levodopa at bedtime may be of benefit if the problem is getting to sleep. However, if this dose does not last the night, sleep may be interrupted. To counter this, another full dose of carbidopa/levodopa can be taken upon awakening in the night. A dose can be laid out on the nightstand with a glass of water, ready to take as needed. As long as at least 3 hours elapse between doses, that should be acceptable. Note that a "full" dose was specified. In other words, use the same dose found optimal during the daytime. Dopamine replenishment for sleep is either very effective or not at all; the dose must reach a threshold amount to work. Intuitively, it may seem that a low dose should be sufficient when one is asleep, but the body does not work that way.

If one is prone to orthostatic hypotension (standing low blood pressure), nighttime levodopa will potentially drop the blood pressure if one needs to get up to use the bathroom. If there is substantial risk of fainting on the way to the washroom, either the nighttime carbidopa/levodopa dose should not be utilized or other strategies for urination should be used, such as a hand-held urinal for men (sitting on the bedside).

Nighttime Urination

The medical term for urination during the night is *nocturia*. General treatment principles for bladder problems were addressed in Chapter 14, which may be worth reviewing. There are a few simple strategies for reducing nocturia although among older adults, it often cannot be entirely eliminated.

Nocturia will be exacerbated if the levodopa coverage during the night is insufficient (see above section). Therefore, adequate nighttime carbidopa/levodopa treatment is advisable.

Nocturia can be reduced by employing a few common-sense strategies:

1. Reduce evening fluids.
2. Urinate right before going to bed.
3. Avoid taking water pills (diuretics) later in the day (morning only).
4. Avoid caffeine beyond late afternoon (a diuretic).

Also, if chronic leg edema (swelling) is ongoing, it may be wise to elevate the legs (to the level of the heart) early in the evening, well before bedtime. This allows gravity to pull the fluid back into the circulation, which can then be eliminated by the kidneys; this translates into urination before going to bed. In other words, for those with chronic edema, lying down has a delayed diuretic effect. Elevation of the legs leads to urination as the leg fluid eventually goes through the kidneys and is converted to urine.

A trip to the bathroom sometimes leads to full awakening and may be disruptive to sleep partners. Alternatives include a bedside commode or, for men, a hand-held urinal at bedside.

Finally, a drug for inhibiting bladder urgency may be tried: trospium. Recall from Chapter 14 that this is the only drug from its class that does not pass into the brain and impair memory. However, it does have other side effects, including dry mouth and eyes, plus constipation. If taken solely for nocturia, trospium may be given as a single 20 mg bedtime dose.

Simple Awakening

Awakening during the night, with trouble returning to sleep, is common in general but especially common among those with DLB and PDD. Simple strategies directed at good sleep hygiene are relevant to this problem, as listed above. Adequate nighttime levodopa coverage should not be overlooked. If all of these recommendations are insufficient, a sleep medicine may be considered. There are two strategies: (1) administration of a longer-acting sleep medicine at bedtime; or (2) taking a short-acting sleep drug upon awakening.

Longer-acting sleep medications taken at bedtime may help consolidate sleep, but if the person is awakened during the night, confusion or unsteadiness may ensue. A routine trip to the bathroom could then become an adventure. See the earlier section "Sedating Antidepressant Drugs" for medications often used to reduce nighttime awakening.

The short-acting sleep drugs generally lose their sedating effect within a few hours, so if they are not taken too close to rising their effect should be gone by morning. Prescription drugs of this type include zolpidem (Ambien), zaleplon (Sonata), and eszopiclone (Lunesta). A dose in the middle of the night should restore sleep. However, there is potential for confusion and imbalance for the next 2 to 4 hours if one is awakened.

Be aware that sleep aids administered during the night could have sedating effects carrying over into the morning. This is true even for the short-acting drugs discussed above.

Nighttime Cramps

Cramps in bed at night are common among most older adults. In those with DLB and PDD, frequent foot, toe, or leg cramps may be a clue to inadequate nighttime levodopa coverage. This may signal loss of the levodopa effect or levodopa underdosage in general. These cramps respond to nocturnal levodopa treatment, outlined in Chapter 9.

INSUFFICIENT TIME SPENT IN BED AT NIGHT

Some people go to bed too late and get up too early. This is a sleep hygiene issue that may be overlooked. It is easy to gradually slip into bad habits. Watching one more show on TV before bed is often a factor. Other people get energized in the evening and dislike retiring before midnight. That pattern may work well in retirement, but not if the alarm continues to be set, or if one is awakened by a spouse who is leaving for work in the early morning. Note that 7 to 9 hours of good sleep is the usual requirement.

POOR-QUALITY SLEEP AT NIGHT (DESPITE ADEQUATE TIME IN BED)

A common cause of daytime drowsiness is failure to achieve adequate deep sleep at night. All people cycle through stages of sleep, going from light sleep to deeper then very deep sleep, and then back to light sleep again. Deep sleep may be prevented by either breathing disruptions (sleep apnea) or intermittent involuntary leg jerks (periodic leg movements of sleep). Each of these disorders is common and should be considered among those who get drowsy during the day.

Sleep Apnea

Sleep apnea implies that breathing becomes impaired during the night. Most often, this relates to the upper airway (back of the throat) collapsing during deep sleep, when the muscles become very relaxed. As soon as this happens, breathing is obstructed. When blood oxygen levels drop, this is sensed by the brain, resulting in a partial arousal to restore adequate breathing. This partial arousal returns the sleeper to a lighter stage of sleep. Consequently, over the course of an entire night, very little deep sleep may occur. Everyone needs deep sleep, and without it people experience daytime drowsiness. This lack of deep sleep may cause other problems as well, such as impaired thinking or elevation of blood pressure, and occasionally it may predispose to serious heart rhythm problems (e.g., atrial fibrillation).

Certain nighttime clues suggest sleep apnea, including loud snoring or interrupted breathing. Body habitus may suggest a potential for this; sleep apnea is more likely among those who are obese, especially those with a thick neck. Sleep apnea seems to be especially common among those with Lewy disorders, although this may reflect the closer scrutiny by clinicians treating DLB and PDD.

Definite diagnosis of sleep apnea is made at a sleep center or clinic. The person being evaluated sleeps overnight with monitoring of various parameters, including brain waves and breathing. This testing is termed polysomnography. Screening for sleep apnea can be done at home with overnight oximetry. The patient receives a digital recording device to take home and places an oxygen sensor on one finger at bedtime. This sensor is similar to the finger oxygen sensors used in the hospital. The finger sensor measures blood oxygen as the person sleeps and digitally records the results, which can be printed out the next day. Oximetry is not fail-proof and it may miss or overcall sleep apnea, so assessment in the sleep laboratory is ultimately necessary if there is clinical suspicion or doubt about the results.

Treatment of sleep apnea is usually very gratifying. The conventional treatment is termed continuous positive airway pressure, or CPAP. It involves a facial mask that fits snugly and administers air pressure to keep the airways open. If the mask is not tolerated there are other strategies as well.

Periodic Limb Movements of Sleep (PLMS)

PLMS are often associated with restless legs syndrome, but sometimes they occur independently. They may be recognized by the sleep partner as intermittent jerks of the legs at night. They are termed periodic because they tend to recur at certain regular intervals, often every 20 to 30 seconds. Typically, the hip will flex and the knee bend, abating after 2 to 3 seconds and then being quiescent for the next half-minute or so. These movements recur intermittently during portions of the night. Like sleep apnea, they may impair deep sleep by causing a mini-arousal so that sleep reverts to a lighter stage with each leg kick. If only a few of these movements occur, a night's sleep may still be adequate. However, if many occur, daytime drowsiness may be the consequence of this loss of deep sleep.

PLMS are often overlooked by the sleep partner and sleeper. The definitive diagnosis can be made during overnight evaluation at a sleep center (polysomnography).

The treatment for PLMS is the same as that for restless legs syndrome: dopamine replenishment (i.e., carbidopa/levodopa). Thus, if a dose of carbidopa/levodopa is being administered at bedtime, this should effectively treat PLMS, at least during the first half of the night. If there is concern that PLMS may be recurring later in the night, another dose of carbidopa/levodopa can be used. Sometimes it may be appropriate to empirically treat the affected person on a trial basis. If sleep quality improves from a bedtime dose of carbidopa/levodopa, it may be useful to continue.

DAYTIME DROWSINESS FROM MEDICATIONS

Medications taken for pain, anxiety, or muscle relaxation tend to induce drowsiness. As mentioned in Chapter 12, they may also impair thinking. Examples of such drugs are listed in Table 16.1.

Quetiapine (Seroquel) is the medication conventionally used in DLB or PDD to treat hallucinations and delusions, but it also induces drowsiness. This is not problematic when this drug is only administered at bedtime, as is the practice with Lewy disorders. When this drug is used for psychosis in other disorders (e.g., schizophrenia), it is administered both morning and night. The morning dose is usually not necessary in DLB or PDD. Another drug used for psychosis that induces drowsiness is clozapine (Clozaril), but it is rarely used because of other side effects.

Table 16.1 Medications that May Induce Drowsiness

Narcotic Pain Medications	Non-Narcotic Pain Medications	Muscle Relaxants	Anxiety Relievers (Primarily Benzodiazepines)
Oxycodone (in Percodan, Oxycontin); hydrocodone (in Vicodin, Lortab); codeine (in Tylenol #3); and others	Tramadol (Ultram, Ultracet); butal- bital (in headache medications)	Tizanidine (Zanaflex); baclofen (Lioresal); cyclobenzaprine (Flexeril); orphenadrine (Norgesic, Norflex); carisop- rodol (Soma); chlorzoxazone (Parafon Forte)	Clonazepam (Klonopin); diaz- epam (Valium); alprazolam (Xanax); lorazepam (Ativan); clorazepate (Tranxene); hydroxyzine (Atarax, Vistaril)

The dopamine agonists may induce sleepiness in a minority of people. These drugs include pramipexole (Mirapex), ropinirole (Requip), and rotigotine (Neupro). With the regular formulations of pramipexole or ropinirole taken three times daily the sleepiness is easy to recognize, since it follows each dose. However, this may be overlooked among those taking the extended-release form of these drugs or the rotigotine patch. With those formulations, the drowsiness is not tightly linked to each dose.

Certain medications taken at bedtime for sleep have long durations of action. Rarely, drowsiness may persist into the following morning. Longer-acting drugs with this potential include clonazepam (Klonopin), diazepam (Valium), flurazepam (Dalmane), amitriptyline, doxepin, and the drugs mentioned for psychosis, quetiapine and clozapine. If morning sleepiness is suspected from a bedtime dose of one of these medications, the patient can experiment by not taking it one night, perhaps substituting a short-acting sleep aid provided by the clinician.

DLB AND PDD: EXCESSIVE SLEEP MAY BE PART OF THE DISORDER

Treatable causes of drowsiness have been the focus of this chapter. However, individuals with DLB or PDD notoriously experience major aberrations of sleep as a component of their Lewy disorder. Sometimes this manifests as sleep attacks: the person simply falls asleep mid-day, for no apparent reason. More concerning to the family and caregivers are the occasional people who intermittently lapse into very prolonged and deep sleep, unable to be aroused. When family members or nursing staff are unable to arouse the person, the worst is assumed. Often this leads to a trip to the emergency room or hospitalization. The true cause may not be apparent until it is recognized as a recurring event, with negative diagnostic studies. A consultation with a sleep specialist is sometimes necessary to clarify what is transpiring.

Lesser states of drowsiness can also be a fundamental part of the sleep disorder seen in DLB or PDD. In this chapter, we have focused on identifying treatable causes. However, if the primary cause is the Lewy condition itself, then there may not be an easy solution. For such problems stimulants are sometimes tried after the workup has turned up no other causative factors.

STIMULANTS

Stimulants are medications that keep people awake. Such drugs are discussed at the end of this chapter because they are a last option and are best deferred until treatable causes of daytime drowsiness have been addressed (such as poor nocturnal sleep and sedating medications).

Stimulants include caffeinated beverages and, most notably, coffee. These are relatively benign and certainly acceptable to use. However, prescription stimulants also deserve special discussion here.

Prescription Stimulants

Prescription stimulants include methylphenidate (Ritalin, Concerta, Daytrana), modafinil (Provigil), and armodafinil (Nuvigil). These drugs are much more effective in countering drowsiness than simple caffeine or coffee. They should be used only after all other treatment strategies for daytime drowsiness have been addressed, including optimizing nighttime sleep and limiting daytime use of sedating medications. Prescription stimulants do have several limitations, including a diminished response with chronic use and the potential for dependence. They may contribute to hallucinations or delusions in susceptible people, and depression may accompany withdrawal. However, they may be very helpful when drowsiness is severe and otherwise untreatable. If used, there should be close follow-up with the prescribing clinician.

Methylphenidate is the oldest of the drugs discussed for this purpose and is also used to treat attention-deficit disorder. The standard pill formulation has a short duration of effect lasting just a few hours, but longer-acting patches and sustained-release formulations are also available. A morning dose of these slow-release forms may impair sleep at bedtime in occasional people.

Modafinil (Provigil) and armodafinil (Nuvigil) are long-acting stimulant drugs taken once each morning. The effect may persist until bedtime and potentially make it difficult to fall asleep. In my experience, the prescription stimulants tend to be effective initially, but have waning benefits with sustained use. Nonetheless, they may be tried after other treatable factors have been addressed.

17

Acting out Dreams

REM Sleep Behavior Disorder

Normal dreaming occurs during the deepest sleep states. Obviously, if experiencing a frightening dream, sleeping people could be injured if they jumped out of bed and started to run. Fortunately, the brain has a natural protective mechanism during dreaming: body paralysis. During the primary sleep stage in which dreaming occurs, the body's muscle tone is shut off and muscles become limp. Only the eye muscles are spared, still able to move during a dream. This state in which dreaming takes place is rapid eye movement (REM) sleep. Restated, during REM sleep, a switch is thrown in the brain stem that shuts off body movement during dreaming.

People with Lewy disorders of all types often lose this switch function. In other words, they can still move during the dreams of REM sleep. In the midst of a dream, they may act out by yelling, kicking, or hitting the air. This behavior is termed dream enactment behavior. When it is a recurring event it is termed REM sleep behavior disorder.

REM sleep behavior disorder occurs in people with Lewy disorders—Parkinson's disease, DLB, or PDD. It also occurs in another disorder in which alpha-synuclein is abnormally deposited in the nervous system, multiple system atrophy (MSA). Recall from Chapter 2 that alpha-synuclein is present in Lewy bodies and is thought to be a causative factor in all of these conditions.

REM sleep behavior disorder may be present years or even decades before the occurrence of DLB, PDD, Parkinson's disease, or multiple system atrophy. It is often one of the first signs of these disorders, predating most other manifestations. That does not mean that everyone who acts out their dreams will eventually develop Parkinson's disease, DLB, or MSA. However, it does confer an increased risk. It should be noted that certain medications may provoke REM sleep behavior disorder, such as the commonly used antidepressants. Also, sleepwalking in children should not be confused with this disorder. Sleepwalking occurs in a different sleep stage and is not thought to be a forerunner of Lewy body conditions.

REM sleep behavior disorder also differs from nighttime sleepwalking and other sleep behaviors occasionally triggered by sedatives such as triazolam (Halcion). People taking these drugs have been known to engage in some very complex behaviors during sleep, such as making trips to the refrigerator.

People with REM sleep behavior disorder do not display this every night and sometimes not even every week or month. There may be long quiescent periods between episodes. The disorder may surface before or after the diagnosis of DLB or Parkinson's disease. There seems to be no relationship between the severity of the Lewy condition and the REM sleep behavior disorder.

IS THIS IMPORTANT?

Sleep specialists have concluded that such dream enactment behavior does not substantially impair sleep quality, unlike sleep apnea or periodic leg movements of sleep, discussed in Chapter 16. Apparently, people with REM sleep behavior disorder still get a good night's sleep, probably because the dream enactment behavior is infrequent; it does not recur often during the night, and it is often quiescent for days or more.

The primary threat is injury risk to the patient or sleep partner. This might occur while running from a villain during a dream, falling out of bed. Similarly, if one is defending against an attacker, the punches might hit the unsuspecting spouse or partner. On a lesser note, frequent yelling or shouting might keep the sleep partner awake.

DO NOT MISINTERPRET

REM sleep behavior disorder should not be misinterpreted as nighttime confusion or hallucinations. How does one distinguish these conditions? People with REM sleep behavior disorder are asleep and will remain asleep unless awakened. They cannot carry on a meaningful conversation. They are responding to whoever or whatever is in their dream, rather than the sleep partner. Conversely, those with DLB or PDD who awaken confused or hallucinating are no longer asleep and can engage in a conversation. They may be mixed up, but a dialogue can be established with the sleep partner.

It is important to distinguish REM sleep behavior disorder from night-time confusional episodes because the treatment is quite different. REM sleep behavior disorder is a much more benign condition. People acting out their dreams do not need to be awakened and do not need protection, except for precautions to prevent injury.

TREATMENT OF REM SLEEP
BEHAVIOR DISORDER

This disorder is treated only if the sleeper is a danger to themselves or a sleep partner. First, the sleep environment should be surveyed; modifications should be made to avoid injury if the sleeper were to fall out of bed or vigorously move around. Sharp corners on nightstands or bedposts should be either padded or removed. Also, it may be appropriate to place a pad next to the bed if a fall onto the floor seems possible.

The sleep partner may also be at risk. For example, if the sleeper is fighting or defending him- or herself in a dream, the sleep partner may be the object of the blows. Obviously, the sleep partner can avoid that by moving to another bed.

Medications are typically effective in controlling REM sleep behavior disorder. The usual medication used for that purpose is clonazepam. This drug is from the Valium class (benzodiazepine) and has side effects of sedation and imbalance. Because it is used as a single dose at bedtime, it usually is well tolerated. One needs to be aware, however, that if awakening to go to the bathroom, clonazepam may cause confusion and a fall risk. The first few times it is used, it is wise for the spouse, partner, or family to be aware of this nighttime risk. On the other hand, clonazepam may also help ensure sounder sleep.

The typical clonazepam dosage is a single 0.5 mg tablet at bedtime. If this is insufficient it may be raised to two tablets at bedtime. Usually that is sufficient, but occasionally the dose may need to be as high as 1.5 to 2 mg before bed. Note that the dream enactment behavior does not need to be completely abolished; rather, it needs to be reduced sufficiently to avoid injuries to the sleeper or the sleep partner. Occasional talking or yelling during sleep does not necessarily need to be treated.

Other drugs from the benzodiazepine class may work similarly; however, they would have the same side effects, so there is no advantage to other drugs from this class.

Over-the-counter melatonin may be helpful in attenuating REM sleep behavior disorder. It can be started as a single 3 mg bedtime dose. If that proves insufficient, it can be raised by 3 mg increments to as high as 12 mg at bedtime. Carbidopa/levodopa does not consistently influence dream enactment behavior.

MORE GENERAL ISSUES

Up to this point in the text, component problems that are notoriously encountered in DLB and PDD have been addressed, focusing especially on treatment. Broader topics that should also be addressed relate to general activities, family, caregivers, and nurses, as well as practical issues such as finances and driving. A person's sense of well-being and affective state are an integral part in all of this, so the discussion begins with depression.

18

Depression

A diagnosis of DLB or PDD might make anyone depressed. It may also depress the spouse and family, although that is a topic for a later chapter. There are several reasons for depression in those with DLB or PDD. First, it may be a reaction to the diagnosis. Second, depression may also be a response to the limitations placed on life and activities. Third, it may reflect Lewy neurodegenerative damage within brain regions that mediate affect. Further complicating this issue is the fact that signs of parkinsonism give the appearance of depression (e.g., masked face). Moreover, symptoms that psychiatrists consider to be vegetative signs of depression, such as apathy, are also common primary symptoms of parkinsonian disorders.

SYMPTOMS AND SIGNS OF DEPRESSION, BUT NOT TRULY DEPRESSED

Depression is a quality-of-life issue that needs attention and appropriate treatment. Recognizing true depression is a crucial starting point and may be difficult in the context of DLB or PDD. Parkinsonian features often make someone appear depressed when clinically they are not. The following are primary symptoms and signs of parkinsonism that may be mis-interpreted as evidence of depression:

- Loss of facial animation (masking)
- Slow to respond (bradykinesia)
- Slowed thinking (bradyphrenia)
- Apathy and loss of motivation
- Poor appetite (sometimes)
- Sleep disorder

Moreover, declining engagement in sports, gardening, yard work, and other activities, may simply be due to the challenges of parkinsonism rather than to depression.

Occasionally, people with DLB or PDD develop *pseudobulbar affect*, which is characterized by a markedly reduced threshold for crying (or laughing) in response to emotional stimuli. For example, mildly emotional stimuli easily provoke tears, such as a religious hymn or ritual. Similarly, scenes in a movie that might bring a tear to the eye of most people provoke uncontrollable crying. People with this condition report incongruity between what they are feeling and the emotional display. Pseudobulbar affect is important to recognize, as this is a component of the neurologic disorder and is not true depression. Although pseudobulbar affect is not true depression, it may respond to a low dose of certain antidepressants: tricyclics (e.g., nortriptyline, amitriptyline) or an SSRI (e.g., fluoxetine, sertraline); see the discussion below of antidepressant drugs.

Clinicians sometimes use depression questionnaires, which generate scores diagnostic of depression. However, these are primarily relevant to people without DLB, PDD, or Parkinson's disease. For example, on the most commonly used depression questionnaire, the primary symptoms of DLB and PDD would lead to affirmative responses on many of these depression questions.

How to Diagnose and Gauge the Severity?

The savvy clinician knows to go beyond first impressions when assessing depression in the setting of DLB or PDD. Talking to both the patient and family is important, as is asking the right questions. Certainly most people with DLB or PDD may well experience at least some depression given the diagnosis and its implications. The challenge to the clinician is to gauge the extent of depression, the need for specific treatment, and the urgency.

Sometimes what initially passes for depression is a loss of interest and a general apathy. This often reflects the decline in motivation that is a component of some Lewy disorders more than of true depression. Apathy rarely responds to treatment with antidepressant drugs or carbidopa/levodopa.

TREATMENT OF DEPRESSION IN DLB AND PDD

Antidepressant medications or psychiatry consultations are not always the first and foremost treatment choice. The clinician's initial formulation is based on the interview with the patient and family. The strategy for addressing possible depression may then be broken down into the following distinctive scenarios.

Patients with Very Dark Thoughts and Suicidal Ideation

This situation demands immediate attention and typically an urgent psychiatric consultation. Fortunately, this is uncommon in these Lewy disorders. If it is present it often leads to admission to the hospital, close monitoring, and aggressive treatment.

Those with Prominent Depression but Who Are Not Suicidal

If the clinician concludes that substantial depression is present but without urgent implications, starting an antidepressant medication is the typical strategy.

The most commonly prescribed antidepressant medications are from the well-known Prozac class. These drugs are categorized as selective serotonin reuptake inhibitors, often abbreviated SSRI. Serotonin is a neurotransmitter (as is dopamine).

Serotonin neurons are primarily within the midline of the brain stem and are thought to be very important in mediating emotions (affect). The SSRI drugs facilitate the actions of serotonin.

The *R* in SSRI stands for reuptake, the process at the synapse where the released neurotransmitter is removed (taken back up). Reuptake terminates its action at the receptor. By blocking its reuptake, serotonin persists in the synapse, prolonging its activity. The antidepressant effect may not be that simple, as it typically takes weeks for the antidepressant benefit to be noticed. However, serotonin facilitation appears to be fundamental to the response.

The SSRIs include various drugs that do not have dramatic differences: fluoxetine (Prozac), sertraline (Zoloft), paroxetine (Paxil), citalopram (Celexa), escitalopram (Lexapro), fluvoxamine (Luvox), and others. They are taken once daily, usually in the morning (if they are sedating they can be taken at bedtime).

A newer class of antidepressants blocks reuptake of not only serotonin but also norepinephrine, which is another neurotransmitter in brain circuits mediating affective (emotional) states; these are termed SSRI/SNRI drugs. This class includes venlafaxine (Effexor), which is started once daily then increased to two to three times daily. It is also available as a once-daily extended-release formulation. The other member of this drug class is duloxetine (Cymbalta), which is taken once daily (occasionally twice daily). These two drugs can have an alerting effect and may interfere with sleep if taken late in the day.

Tricyclic antidepressants are an older class of medications for treating depression. They are as effective at treating depression as the newer SSRI/SNRI drugs but have more side effects. They are also reuptake inhibitors, targeting serotonin, norepinephrine, or dopamine, depending on the drug. These drugs variably tend to induce sleepiness (antihistamine effect) and are administered once daily at bedtime. As discussed in

Chapter 16, low doses may be used as a sleep aid. Drugs in this class include amitriptyline (Elavil), nortriptyline (Pamelor, Aventyl), imipramine (Tofranil), desipramine (Norpramin), doxepin (Sinequan), trimipramine (Surmontil), and protriptyline (Surmontil). Besides sleepiness, these drugs also have anticholinergic properties, to varying degrees. As discussed in previous chapters, drugs that block acetylcholine (i.e., anticholinergics) tend to be constipating, slow urination, produce dry the mouth and eyes, and may impair memory.

Two other commonly used antidepressant drugs that do not fall into the above classes are mirtazapine (Remeron) and bupropion (Wellbutrin). Mirtazapine is very sedating and is taken once daily at bedtime; it may be particularly beneficial for those who also experience insomnia. Bupropion predominantly blocks reuptake of dopamine (in contrast to the SSRI drugs, which block reuptake of serotonin). It is taken two to three times daily. One might think that bupropion would be the best choice for those with a brain dopamine deficiency typical of DLB and PDD. Arguably, however, bupropion influences on brain dopamine might be overshadowed by carbidopa/levodopa therapy. There have been no comparative studies of any of these agents in the setting of DLB or PDD.

Obviously, many drugs are available as options for depression treatment. No particular one has surfaced as clearly superior. The choice is often based on side effects; however, side effects sometimes are advantageous, such as sedation for someone who experiences insomnia.

People with Non-Disabling Depression

Depression does not always need to be treated with antidepressant drugs. Moreover, these drugs have limitations: (1) they do not help every depressed patient; (2) the antidepressant benefits are often only partial; (3) they have side effects. Hence, for those whose depression is not severe, other strategies may be considered, at least initially.

Treatment of parkinsonism with carbidopa/levodopa.

This medical option should not be overlooked as an effective treatment for mild depressive symptoms. It may help in more than one way. First, adequate levodopa coverage often extends the capacity to engage in activities. Second, replenishment of dopamine may have a primary antidepressant effect. Note that the antidepressant effect of certain drugs discussed earlier, such as desipramine and bupropion, is attributed to facilitating brain dopamine transmission (i.e., blocking reuptake of dopamine). Improvement of dopamine neurotransmission may itself have an antidepressant effect.

Exercise.

The antidepressant effect of physical (aerobic) exercise is substantial. After a vigorous workout or strenuous yard work, the salience of emotionally charged issues tends to diminish. There is also reason to believe that aerobic exercise directly benefits brain function. Regular engagement in an active exercise routine should not be overlooked as an effective and inexpensive strategy for dealing with depression and other psychological problems.

Those with DLB and PDD may have substantial exercise limitations, so enabling the person's engagement in regular exercise may require some creative ideas from family members and caregivers. This topic is discussed further in Chapter 20.

A good balance between novelty and familiarity.

Most of us like new and novel activities and events. Going to a new restaurant or visiting another city is exciting and uplifting. However, people with cognitive impairment (DLB, PDD) may do poorly in new environments, perhaps because very novel surroundings can be confusing, intimidating, and overwhelming. Thus, eating out may be enjoyed if a familiar restaurant is chosen. The balance between novelty and familiarity differs from person to person and may change over time. Observant families and caregivers will need to find the appropriate balance for their loved one with PDD or DLB.

Sleep.

Adequate sleep is a very helpful treatment for depression. Although insomnia is well recognized as a symptom of depression in the general population, it may have separate causes among those with DLB and PDD. Treating insomnia and correcting sleep deprivation should facilitate treatment of depression(discussed in Chapters 9 and 16).

Talk therapy.

Depressed people are often directed to therapists to talk out their problems. This may be appropriate for some with DLB or PDD, but less so among those with prominent cognitive impairment.

OTHER MEDICATION ISSUES

Drug Interactions, Selegiline, Rasagiline

As discussed in Chapter 5, it is sensible to simplify the medication regimen for those individuals with DLB and PDD. The more anti-Parkinson drugs being taken, the greater the likelihood of hallucinations or delusions. Occasionally, however, people are left on selegiline or rasagiline (MAO-B inhibitors) if these are being tolerated. These two drugs have been designated as contraindicated with nearly all the antidepressant medications. The risk of a serious interaction is very small, and most clinicians do not regard this as a substantial risk, provided there is a good indication for both drugs. For those with DLB or PDD who are taking selegiline or rasagiline, it may be wise to discuss the potential risk with the clinician before initiating an antidepressant medication. Because of the long duration of action of both of these drugs, selegiline and rasagiline may be abruptly discontinued.

SSRI Drugs and Parkinsonism

Around the time the SSRI drugs were first introduced, several reports documented worsening of parkinsonism in patients with Parkinson's disease. There has now been a wealth of experience with these drugs in the setting of Parkinson's disease, as well as in DLB and PDD, and the risk of aggravating parkinsonism appears to be minimal. These medications are commonly used to treat depression in people with DLB or PDD.

*Electrocardiographic changes from
excessive doses of SSRI drugs.*

The SSRI drugs should be used in the dosages stipulated by the clinician, and not raised unless advised to do so. A serious cardiac rhythm disturbance, prolonged QT syndrome, can be provoked by very high doses of SSRI drugs.

ELECTROCONVULSIVE THERAPY (ECT)

ECT involves induction of a brain seizure by a single shock to the head. This method sounds barbaric and is used only rarely for the most serious and treatment-refractory of psychiatric problems. Severe depression that fails other treatments is one of those conditions that may lend itself to ECT. It is the rare person with DLB or PDD in whom this is considered appropriate, but in the right situation it can restore a life. It does not impair control of parkinsonism, and parkinsonism actually improves for a few days after an ECT session. Confusion typically worsens for a few days but this is transient. ECT is reserved for desperate problems. In the right circumstance, the outcome can be very gratifying.

19

General Medical Issues

People with DLB and PDD tend to be middle-aged and older. In this age group, selected general health issues deserve discussion. Comprehensive medical care is beyond the scope of this book, but several general medical topics should be addressed here.

FALLS AND OSTEOPOROSIS

People with Lewy disorders commonly experience walking difficulties. The risk of falling may surface early or later in the condition. Fracture risk is also a concern, and preemptive action is wise. Falls can be tolerated if bones are strong; witness athletes who fall on a football field.

Over the course of a lifetime, bones tend to lose their strength and become more prone to fractures. When the loss of bone integrity is substantial we categorize this as osteoporosis. There are specific criteria that doctors use to define osteoporosis. While bone integrity is measured in several ways, the most common and accepted measurement is by imaging with a nuclear medicine technique. A quick scan after injection of a radioisotope that is taken up by bones generates a picture and numeric data; these can be compared to those of normal subjects. This analysis is termed a nuclear medicine bone density study and sometimes is called a DEXA scan.

Using the numeric measures from a bone density scan, reductions of bone integrity fall into two classes. We have already mentioned that substantial loss of bone strength is termed *osteoporosis*. A less severe reduction of bone integrity has been defined and termed *osteopenia*. Restated, mild bone weakening is osteopenia, and marked loss of bone integrity is osteoporosis.

Conventionally, osteoporosis is treated with prescription medications, whereas the lesser problem of osteopenia is not. However, if there is a substantial fall risk, some clinicians would advise treating osteopenia with a prescription drug (see below).

Who is at risk for osteoporosis? In the general population, advancing age is the major risk factor. Women over age 60 and men over age 70 fall into these risk categories, as well as those with very sedentary lives. In the context of DLB or PDD, osteoporosis is especially important to consider.

General Treatment

Two conditions that exacerbate bone weakening and lead to osteoporosis are calcium deficiency and inactivity. Each is treatable, and osteoporosis due to these problems is at least partially preventable.

Our body needs an ongoing supply of calcium in the circulation and in the fluids in and around the organs. It is crucial to normal nerve, muscle, and brain function. The body has a finely tuned system for maintaining stable calcium levels. If the circulating calcium in the bloodstream declines, hormones are activated that release it from bones. Bones are full of calcium and are the calcium reservoir for the body. However, pulling calcium out of bones necessarily weakens them. A strategy for avoiding this is to maintain adequate intake of calcium in the diet.

Adequate vitamin D is crucial for calcium absorption from the gut. While vitamin D supplementation has been advocated for a variety of disorders, current evidence has only proven the benefits for bone health and calcium absorption. Future research may suggest other roles for vitamin D.

Recently, there has been much discussion in the medical literature about the optimum amount of calcium and vitamin D in our diets and supplements. A fairly conservative and acceptable recommendation from a combination of diet and supplements each day is as follows:

1200 mg of calcium
800 to 1000 units of vitamin D

These are appropriate recommendations for all adults.

Clinicians are well aware that nonuse of a limb (e.g., casting) will leave the bones weaker and less dense on X-ray. Conversely, use of a limb against some resistive force tends to strengthen bones, or at least prevent bone weakening. Therefore, a sedentary lifestyle tends to facilitate osteoporosis, whereas exercise has the opposite effect. Exercise is important to maintaining bone integrity, and aerobic exercise also benefits brain function, as outlined in Chapter 20.

Specific Treatment of Osteoporosis

Once osteoporosis is diagnosed with the nuclear medicine (DEXA) scan it is typically treated with a prescription medication. The most common class of drugs is the bisphosphonates, which include alendronate (Fosamax), risedronate (Actonel, Atelvia), zoledronic acid (Reclast, Zometa), and ibandronate (Boniva). Other drugs for addressing osteoporosis include the bone hormone analogue, teriparatide (Forteo), and the female hormone drug, raloxifene (Evista). The appropriate choice is made by the clinician.

DIET, VITAMINS, AND WEIGHT

Is a Special Diet Advisable?

There has been a plethora of special diets advocated for treatment of nearly every medical condition. Should individuals with Lewy disorders have a special diet? The simple answer is no, but a few common sense principles should be addressed.

First, if the person is taking carbidopa/levodopa, it should be separated from meals, as discussed in Chapter 6. Digested protein from our meals liberates the constituent amino acids. These dietary amino acids compete with levodopa for transport into the brain. However, the diet does not need to be changed, as long as the carbidopa/levodopa doses are at least 1 hour before and at least 2 hours after the end of meals.

North American diets often contain high concentrations of saturated fats and trans-fats. These can promote atherosclerosis. For general health reasons, it is wise to limit such fats and to liberally consume fruits and vegetables.

North American diets also tend to be high in calories, often exceeding the daily caloric expenditure (i.e., we take in more calories than we burn with exercise). Individuals with Lewy disorders with the inherent gait and balance problems suffer in the face of obesity. Carrying extra body weight makes all movement more difficult. Those with Lewy conditions should try to achieve close to their ideal body weight and avoid obesity. Obesity is an added challenge to caregivers assisting with activities of daily living .

Conventional advice to the general public promotes salt restriction. This has one important purpose in the general population: reduction of blood pressure. This is also an appropriate goal in the context of Lewy disorders, but not so if orthostatic hypotension is present. In the face of low blood pressures, salt intake may be advisable (discussed in detail in Chapter 13).

Vitamins and Supplements

Many older adults self-medicate with various vitamins and health supplements. However, many of these are unnecessary, and some are quite expensive.

What about a conventional multivitamin? In the previous section, vitamin D was discussed as being important for bone health. A typical multivitamin has 400 units of vitamin D, which is around half of the daily requirement. Hence, a multivitamin is useful unless vitamin D is being supplied by other supplements or diet. What about the other ingredients in a multivitamin? It turns out that adequate amounts of these other vitamins are present in typical North American diets. One should not need a vitamin supplement (other than vitamin D and calcium, discussed above) if eating well-balanced meals and provided that the body weight is stable and there are no medical conditions compromising nutrition.

Weight loss may justify an additional vitamin supplement, and a consultation with a dietician is advisable if the loss of weight is more than a few pounds. If substantial weight loss occurs in the absence of dieting, the clinician will need to consider the cause, such as malabsorption or cancer. Weight loss is sometimes associated with DLB and PDD, but it is prudent to not jump to that conclusion.

Selective deficiencies of vitamin B12 or copper occasionally develop in otherwise normal people with good nutrition. Clinicians are aware of this and can measure these substances when they do routine blood work. Deficiencies of vitamin B12 or copper often become apparent with tingling in the feet. With progression of the deficiency, various other neurologic symptoms may develop. For those with such deficiencies, lifelong supplementation is often necessary.

Vitamin supplementation if taking carbidopa/levodopa.

Carbidopa/levodopa treatment may be associated with relative deficits of vitamin B12, vitamin B6, or folic acid. This issue surfaced several years ago when it was documented that people taking carbidopa/levodopa tended to have elevated levels of a blood product, homocysteine. This was recognized to be a consequence of normal levodopa metabolism by the enzyme catechol-O-methyltransferase (COMT). Levodopa metabolism by this enzyme requires the cofactors vitamin B12, vitamin B6, and folic acid, as does normal homocysteine metabolism. If there are not enough of these three vitamins to go around, then blood homocysteine is not adequately metabolized and the levels rise. Could this be a problem? To answer that question, we need to digress and look at the broader issue of homocysteine metabolism in general.

Long before we knew about the association between carbidopa/levodopa and elevated homocysteine levels, scientists noted that elevated blood homocysteine levels were associated with strokes, heart attacks, and dementia. In other words, those in the general population with elevated blood homocysteine concentrations (not taking carbidopa/levodopa) were at a significantly higher risk of later developing a stroke, having a heart attack, or becoming demented. It was also found that high blood homocysteine levels are easily normalized by administering large amounts of folic acid and vitamins B6 and B12. This finding suggested that people at risk for strokes, heart attacks, or dementia might benefit from such vitamin supplementation. Clinical trials have not borne this out; vitamin supplementation has not changed clinical outcomes. It continues to be debated whether the high blood homocysteine levels associated with strokes, heart attacks, and dementia are simply coincidental rather than causative.

What does this mean for people on carbidopa/levodopa treatment? Carbidopa/levodopa raises homocysteine levels, but it is unclear if that is clinically important. It is easy to lower homocysteine levels with the standard three-vitamin pill developed precisely for that purpose, with conventional concentrations:

Vitamin B12 (cyanocobalamin): 2 mg (2000 micrograms [mcg])
Vitamin B6 (pyridoxine): 25 mg
Folic acid: 2.5 mg

A cautious approach for those taking carbidopa/levodopa would be to either measure the homocysteine concentrations in the bloodstream, including whenever the dose is substantially raised, or, alternatively, take the above combination vitamin. The downside of the vitamin is the expense (it is a prescription pill); however, it has no toxicity or side effects. Very high doses of vitamin B6 can result in serious neurologic problems, but that is with doses many times higher than that contained in this pill. Only a small minority of neurologists prescribe this vitamin to their Parkinson's disease patients taking carbidopa/levodopa; however, it is defensible. It is prescribed once daily as the generic but comes in a variety of brand names, such as Foltx, Folbic, Folbee, and Folgard.

Coenzyme Q$_{10}$

Coenzyme Q$_{10}$ is an important biochemical cofactor in mitochondria. Mitochondria are present in all human cells and are crucial for cellular energy production. This is where dietary nutrient products interact with oxygen to produce high-energy molecules fundamental to many body biochemical processes.

Scientists have recognized that mitochondria perform suboptimally in some Lewy disorders, notably Parkinson's disease. Exactly what causative role dysfunctional mitochondria play in these conditions remains unknown.

Since mitochondrial function is impaired in Parkinson's disease, the mitochondrial factor coenzyme Q$_{10}$ has been tried as treatment. The first study, published a decade ago, compared three coenzyme Q$_{10}$ doses to a placebo (sugar pill). Benefit in this small study was noted only in the group receiving the highest amount of coenzyme Q$_{10}$: 1200 mg daily; the lesser doses (300, 600 mg daily) had no apparent benefit. Unfortunately, these results could not be replicated in two larger investigations assessing even higher coenzyme Q$_{10}$ doses. Currently, there appears to be insufficient evidence for coenzyme Q$_{10}$ administration in Parkinson's disease or any Lewy condition such as DLB or PDD. It is expensive in higher doses, although appears to be safe.

OTHER GENERAL HEALTH FACTORS

It is not known what drives the development of Lewy pathology in the nervous system. However, brain vascular health is important since brain atherosclerosis can be additive with Lewy pathology. Atherosclerosis, formerly called hardening of the arteries, is the primary process that underlies strokes and heart attacks. Atherosclerosis involves the buildup of plaque and related material inside the walls of arteries, narrowing the lumen where blood must flow. Such atherosclerosis is not confined to only the larger arteries that become plugged in strokes and heart attacks. In the brain, small arteries in all regions are similarly susceptible. The cumulative atherosclerotic involvement of tiny vessels, apparent on MRI brain scans, may contribute to brain dysfunction. When it involves brain pathways (white matter) it is termed *leukoariosis*. Leukoariosis is typically present to a mild degree with normal aging but is exacerbated by atherosclerotic processes. People with long-standing very high blood pressure or poorly controlled diabetes mellitus tend to have more prominent leukoariosis. Sometimes prominent leukoariosis is well tolerated without obvious neurologic deficits. However, if combined with a Lewy neurodegenerative condition (e.g., DLB or PDD), this may be an additive insult to the brain.

It is wise not to ignore atherosclerotic risk factors. The primary care clinician or internist is in a good position to advise about blood pressure management, cholesterol, and blood sugar (glucose), which are all potential risk factors for atherosclerosis.

Parenthetically, blood pressure is unconsciously controlled by the autonomic nervous system. As discussed in earlier chapters, the autonomic nervous system may be affected in Lewy conditions. The blood pressure problem of Lewy disorders, however, is orthostatic hypotension (Chapter 13), with low readings occurring when a person is up and about.

Exercise

A frequently overlooked contributor to overall health is exercise. In the next chapter, the evidence for aerobic exercise benefiting the brain is reviewed. However, it is also important for general health. Exercise helps combat atherosclerosis. It helps reverse the progressive reduction in muscle bulk due to aging, known as sarcopenia. As discussed earlier, it improves the strength of bones, tending to counter osteoporosis. Exercise also helps fight obesity; carrying extra weight makes all movement more difficult. Exercise also has important psychological benefits, reducing anxiety and countering depression.

20

Benefits of Regular Exercise

Disease-Slowing?

Our culture has seen a generational shift in activity levels. In the 1950s everyone walked. How do I know? I grew up in the 1950s. Cars were typically reserved for day trips or vacations, except for people living in the country. Garages had one stall. Shopping malls had not proliferated and people walked to stores; children did not take buses to school, except for farm kids. Snow was removed with shovels, and grass was cut with push mowers. In a half-century, this scene has changed and we have adopted a sedentary lifestyle. Further contributing to this lifestyle is the proliferation of video games, multichannel TVs with remote controls, and computers. Blue collar work is increasingly done overseas.

A sedentary culture should favor those with DLB or PDD, right? Lewy-related parkinsonism is physically challenging. With our cultural change, there is no longer a need to get up from the chair and walk very far. In fact, a lift chair with a motor will make it easy to stand. Ostensibly, this is all good. However, there is a dark side to this scenario, which is the focus of this chapter. As you have probably already surmised, we are going to enlarge on that old adage "if you don't use it, you lose it." It turns out that there is much truth in that statement, documented in scientific and medical journals.

VIGOROUS EXERCISE AS TREATMENT

Exercising is easy when one is young and energetic, but it becomes increasingly difficult in middle age; it is downright hard during senior years, even with no neurologic or orthopedic conditions. Excuses and alternatives can easily sidetrack the best of intentions. Anything this difficult needs a compelling rationale. This chapter will summarize the scientific evidence suggesting that vigorous exercise has a biological effect on the brain that may well counter neurodegeneration and brain aging.

What Is Vigorous Exercise?

The term *exercise* is used in a variety of ways. In this chapter, the focus is on aerobic exercise, which will also be referred to as vigorous exercise. This is exercise sufficient to induce sweating and raise the heart rate. It differs from stretching and balance exercises that are typically a part of routine physical therapy. Those exercises are important but fundamentally different from aerobic exercise.

Clinicians and scientists studying aerobic exercise measure *fitness*. To do this, they may have the subject peddle a stationary bicycle or run on a treadmill while the amount of oxygen uptake is measured. The person is encouraged to push their exercise performance to the maximum, and at that point, the oxygen uptake is measured. This oxygen uptake at maximum (peak) exercise is used as the measure of fitness. People who are indeed physically fit efficiently take up oxygen; that is to say, they have high levels of measured oxygen as testimony to their fitness. Physiologists term this measure VO_2 at peak exercise (peak VO_2), which is universally employed as a measure of fitness.

To reiterate, the focus here is not on balance training or stretching, which have their own benefits. This chapter addresses benefits of vigorous exercise—that is, exercise that elicits perspiration and makes a person tired.

Is There One Specific Exercise Routine that Is Best?

The lay press has often written about the merits of one specific exercise or another being good for health. However, the exercise advocated here can be accomplished through a vast array of physical activity. Think about all the physical choices available to provoke sweating, fatigue, and raise the heart rate. Going to the gym is one outlet, but so is walking in the neighborhood, especially at a brisk pace. Doing yard work such as raking leaves, pushing a mower, or shoveling dirt are also good outlets. Sit-ups and push-ups on the floor count, as does riding a stationary bicycle in the basement or swimming laps at the YMCA. Individuals with poor balance or bad knees can also find exercise outlets; most workout centers have numerous machines where the exercises can be done sitting. Resistance exercises, when done repeatedly and without much rest, generate good aerobic exercise.

The crucial factor is choice of exercise routines that are doable for the specific individual, but not so onerous that they will be abandoned. Remember that vigorous exercise is not supposed to be easy. It is unrealistic, however, to expect that everyone should become a marathon athlete. Rather, each person should do their best with the hand they are dealt, starting with low levels of exercise and building on that, choosing routines that meet capabilities and are sustainable.

How Can We Prove Exercise Slows the Course of DLB and PDD?

In a perfect world, this hypothesis would be tested with a large multiyear study assessing whether regular aerobic exercise slows the progression of Lewy disorders (i.e., less parkinsonism and better cognition). Voluntary subjects with early DLB or PDD would be randomly allocated to one of two treatments: regular aerobic exercise or a sedentary lifestyle, continuing for perhaps 5 years. At the end of the study, the two groups would be compared on measures of gait, movement, and cognition.

Unfortunately, this study is neither practical nor doable. Some in the exercise group would give up; conversely, some in the sedentary group would recognize the benefits of exercise and workout. Finally, many would simply drop out because of the necessary length of this trial (years) or because of comorbid age-related afflictions (e.g., cancer). Dropouts make clinical trials impossible to interpret, especially if there is disproportionate participation from one group. The remaining subjects may be those with inherently milder disease, biasing results toward a better outcome. Further confounding interpretation would be differing use of neurologic drugs (e.g., carbidopa/levodopa). One could not force the subjects to remain on the same drugs for the duration of the trial. Some would argue that without this perfect clinical trial, skepticism about the benefit of exercise is necessary; however, such a trial will never be done.

Although there is no one perfect clinical trial assessing this issue, there is a wealth of scientific evidence arguing for a disease-slowing benefit from aerobic exercise. Rather than coming from one or a few ideal clinical trials, the evidence comes from many perspectives and many investigations. Nearly all of these point to the conclusion that aerobic exercise has favorable effects on the brain, with the potential to slow neurodegenerative processes and brain aging.

Every point made in this chapter is based on a wealth of studies from peer-reviewed medical and scientific journal articles. The published references substantiating the contents of this chapter are found in two recent review papers written for clinicians:

Ahlskog JE. Does vigorous exercise have a neuroprotective effect in Parkinson disease? *Neurology*, 2011; 77:288–294.

Ahlskog JE, Geda, YE, Graff-Radford, NR, Petersen, RC. Physical exercise as a preventive or disease-modifying treatment of dementia and brain aging. *Mayo Clinic Proceedings*, 2011; 86(9):876–884.A summary of this evidence follows.

EVIDENCE FOR AEROBIC EXERCISE IMPROVING THE COURSE OF LEWY DISORDERS

As already discussed, a perfect clinical experiment to test this hypothesis is impractical. Hence, a more indirect approach is appropriate, which incorporates studies from all perspectives, in humans and animals. Although DLB and PDD are the narrow focus of this book, it is appropriate to take a more a more expansive view and include the scientific literature relating to the influence of exercise on dementia and cognition, in general, as well as that pertaining to Parkinson's disease. Taking these broader views allows a very interesting perspective on the brain benefits of aerobic exercise.

Studies in Humans: Multiple Clinical Trials Summarized by Meta-Analyses

Many topics in medicine have been studied in more than a single clinical trial. If these clinical experiments all generated exactly the same outcome, then the interpretation would be simple. However, chance variation influences all outcomes in science; hence, clinical trials often generate different findings. Medical statisticians have a useful strategy of combining similar clinical trials to evaluate the aggregate outcome, termed *meta-analysis*.

Exercise effects on a variety of brain measures have been studied in many clinical trials. Published meta-analyses of these trials allow interpretation of the aggregate outcomes. We will try to take a balanced view of this published literature, summarizing each set of studies.

Exercise and cognition in the general population.

Many published studies have analyzed the effect of exercise on various aspects of thinking and memory (cognition). An array of studies in normal adults has documented improved cognitive scores after exercise. A meta-analysis of studies in which subjects were randomized to exercise or sedentary activities documented modest but significant benefits; the duration of exercise in these studies ranged from 1 to 18 months. In several other studies, physically fit older adults had significantly better cognitive test scores than those of unfit older adults (fitness measured by oxygen uptake at peak exercise, VO_2).

Numerous studies have tabulated the subsequent risk of dementia among people who exercised and those who did not in mid-life. The meta-analysis revealed a significantly reduced risk of later becoming demented associated with mid-life exercise. Similarly, the risk of later developing mild cognitive impairment was similarly reduced among those who exercised (documented in all five studies).

Magnetic resonance imaging (MRI) of the brain has also shown benefits of exercise in normal people. In such studies, functional MRI was used to document specific brain regions or connections activated by specific tasks. An exercise program lasting 6 to 12 months led to improved functional MRI brain scan results: better cortex connectivity and activation. In another study using functional MRI brain scans, older adults who were physically fit had better cortex activation and connectivity than that in unfit counterparts.

Finally, people who were already experiencing cognitive decline were randomized to an exercise program versus a sedentary lifestyle. The exercise group had significantly improved cognitive scores, in comparison to those with a sedentary lifestyle. This result was replicated in three independent trials.

Brain volumes influenced by exercise.

The normal brain shrinks with age. Scientists have concluded that this primarily relates to a reduction of brain connections, although loss of brain cells makes a small contribution. Neurologists can easily distinguish the MRI brain scan of a normal 80-year-old from that of a 30-year-old. Such reduction in brain volume might contribute to neurologic decline.

The three-dimensional volume of selected brain regions has been studied, including the hippocampus, which is a memory center. The hippocampus is a small region in the temporal lobes of the brain. If the brain's two hippocampi (right and left) are destroyed, new memories cannot be made. With normal aging the hippocampus shrinks. Studies at the University of Illinois have documented remarkable effects of exercise on hippocampal volumes. They have shown a significant relationship between the size of the hippocampus and degree of fitness (peak VO_2); older adults who were more fit had larger hippocampi. This finding was extended in a prospective study of older adults whose hippocampal volumes were measured after a prospective exercise program and compared with those of a control group engaging in a stretching and toning program (nonaerobic exercise). The aerobic exercise group gradually increased the size of their hippocampi over the year of the study, compared to the control group, whose hippocampal volume declined.

The volume of the brain cortex has also been measured before and after a 6-month exercise program in two other studies (see Chapter 4, Figures 4.1 and 4.8, for pictures of the cortex). Small but significant increases in cortical volume were linked to exercise, compared to a sedentary group. Two other investigations documented less age-related cortical volume loss among physically fit older adults, compared to those who were unfit. In yet another study, the distances that people regularly walked were tabulated in mid-life and then assessed 9 years later. Walking distances were subsequently associated with greater volumes of cortex and a reduced risk of cognitive impairment (i.e., walkers had larger cortical volumes and were less likely to experience cognitive decline).

Another Lewy disorder: Parkinson's disease.

Parkinson's disease is the prototypic Lewy disorder. Four prospective studies assessed the risk of later developing Parkinson's disease as a function of mid-life exercise. In these studies, people regularly exercising in mid-life ultimately had a significantly lower risk of later developing Parkinson's disease, compared to those exercising little (confirmed by meta-analysis). Of course, this could simply reflect a disinclination to exercise as a very early symptom of Parkinson's disease (present years before actually manifesting Parkinson's disease).

Does exercise in the setting of Parkinson's disease reduce the later risk becoming demented? This has not been assessed in a well-controlled trial.

Animal Studies

Nearly all animal exercise investigations have been done using rats or mice. Rats and mice will voluntarily run for long periods each day if their home cage contains a running wheel. They will also run on a treadmill. For the purposes of testing, experimenters can prevent use of a limb with a soft restraining cast. Hence, rats and mice are good subjects for exercise experiments.

Many studies in rats and mice have documented better cognitive outcomes with exercise. These animals learn trails in mazes better after exercise; exercised animals learn better than their nonexercised mates. In a single study in monkeys, those engaging in 5 months of regular exercise had better cognitive outcomes, compared to monkeys randomized to a sedentary lifestyle.

A common paradigm for studying experimental parkinsonism in rats or mice is to inject a toxin that selectively destroys the dopamine-containing substantia nigra region (illustrated in Figure 4.4 in Chapter 4). There are two neurotoxins commonly used for that purpose: (1) 6-hydroxydopamine (6-OH-DA), which is injected directly into the nigrostriatal brain region; and (2) MPTP, which is injected into the gut area and travels to the brain, where it destroys the dopamine-containing substantia nigra neurons. In humans, no such toxins are thought to cause Parkinson's disease or other Lewy conditions, but in animals these toxins produce movement problems that are similar to those in Parkinson's disease.

The influence of exercise on the neurologic deficits caused by 6-OH-DA or MPTP has been extensively studied. Exercise reverses the parkinsonism provoked by 6-OH-DA (five of six studies), as well as MPTP (four studies). Conversely, immobilizing a limb so it cannot move exacerbates the neurologic deficits (one study each: 6-OH-DA, MPTP, respectively). In many of these studies, investigators also documented reduced neurotoxin damage to the targeted brain neurons in exercised animals.

Why Should Exercise Counter Potent Neurotoxins?

A vast array of studies have investigated the biochemical changes in the brain that occur with aerobic exercise. Numerous mechanisms for improving brain connections and reversing potential deficits have been documented. Most notable has been the discovery that exercise releases certain brain trophic (growth) factors: brain-derived neurotrophic factor (BDNF) and glial-derived neurotrophic factor (GDNF). This includes release of these substances in the same regions where MPTP and 6-OH-DA are destructive.

Additional studies have assessed the generation of other factors and mechanisms that favor neuroplasticity. Neuroplasticity connotes the generation of new brain connections that are the foundations for memory and learning; they tend to offset age-related brain atrophy. Exercise in animals increases genes and gene products that facilitate neuroplasticity and thus the development of new synaptic connections. The electrical correlate of learning that is studied by scientists is termed long-term potentiation; this also is enhanced by exercise.

WHAT SHOULD WE CONCLUDE FROM THIS?

The totality of the scientific data certainly seems to suggest that regular aerobic exercise is good for the brain and could improve the course of neurodegenerative diseases, including DLB and PDD. This is not proven, but this evidence certainly seems compelling.

How much should one exercise? Where is the point of diminishing returns? The scientific literature does not adequately address this question. One might infer from the studies summarized above that the more fit, the better. However, the fitness of a young athlete is not realistic for many older adults. In the next section, practical strategies to promote exercise will be discussed.

WHAT TO DO

These studies advocate for aerobic exercise, which is physical exercise sufficient to increase heart rate and make one sweat. If continued, it should ultimately result in fitness, although marked fitness may not be realistic for everyone.

Fitness, or at least better fitness, does not occur overnight. It is wise to start with limited exercise routines and realistic goals. The exercise should be gradually increased over months, guided by the body's increasing capacity to perform.

For sedentary individuals, consultation with their internist or primary care physician is often appropriate to make sure that there are no contraindications to a vigorous exercise routine. Consulting with the doctor is mandatory if exercise results in chest pain or if shortness of breath is triggered by modest exercise.

Orthopedic conditions (e.g., painful arthritic knees) or imbalance should not prevent aerobic exercise. Health clubs and gyms have a vast array of exercise machines that allow sitting aerobic exercises. These can be varied to prevent doing the same thing repeatedly. Swimming laps is good exercise that does not put stress on joints.

Brisk walks or jogging is a common form of aerobic exercise. In cold weather climates this can be extended through the winter months by using gyms or walking in enclosed shopping malls.

How much exercise is sufficient? While this has not been adequately studied in clinical trials, the American Heart Association guidelines seem appropriate here (Nelson et al., *Circulation* 2007; 116:1094–1105). They advise "moderate-intensity aerobic physical activity for a minimum of 30 minutes on five days each week or vigorous-intensity aerobic activity for a minimum of 20 minutes on three days each week." To this regimen they also suggest adding resistance exercises at least two days weekly. Resistance exercise involves pushing, pulling, or other effort against resistance on an exercise machine or with free weights.

Is there a limit to how much exercise is desirable? Is more always better? This is unknown and has not been adequately studied. Certainly, older adults should stop short of injuring themselves or making themselves miserable. However, once they have gotten used to the routine at lower exercise levels, they may gently push themselves with an ultimate goal of getting as fit as possible. It may be wise to consult a physical therapist from time to time to get an objective view of how things are progressing. For individuals who are otherwise healthy, a physical trainer may serve the same purpose. There should be a general understanding that fitness is a long-term goal (perhaps achieved in a year or two) and not something that needs to be quickly accomplished.

For those with prominent parkinsonism as part of DLB, the guidelines for initiating and escalating carbidopa/levodopa treatment, discussed in Chapter 6, are important to know and implement. Exercise is difficult in the face of untreated parkinsonism. It makes sense to treat the parkinsonism first, optimizing the carbidopa/levodopa dosage, and then begin the exercise program.

OTHER BENEFITS OF REGULAR EXERCISE

This chapter has focused on benefits to the brain. In addition, there are other well-accepted exercise benefits to health in general. Cardiologists recommend exercise to maintain good heart and circulatory function. Doctors treating stroke take the same view. Along these same lines, atherosclerosis risk factors improve with regular exercise, including blood pressure and lipid control. Diabetics similarly benefit from exercise, which not only decreases other risk factors but also favors glucose control.

An important component of osteoporosis prevention and treatment is regular exercise. Exercise helps counter the age-related trend toward sarcopenia (atrophy of muscles). Depression and anxiety also improve with regular exercise.

Maintaining an ideal body weight facilitates longevity, and exercise is an important component of such a program. In fact, one recent study linked regular exercise with longer lifespans.

FINAL THOUGHTS

Common sense should always be brought to bear on any medical recommendation. Before starting a new exercise program, be sure the primary care doctor approves of it. Start with modest goals. If unfamiliar with exercise routines, engage a physical therapist and emphasize that an active aerobic exercise program is desired (i.e., not just stretching and doing balance exercises, although those are also important). Listen to the body and modify the routine to accommodate problematic joints and limbs. If knees are painful, choose exercises that can be done sitting and that do not require abusing those joints. If able, consider swimming laps. Finally, if exercise provokes new heart or lung symptoms, stop, and inform the physician. Although it may be good to work through some minor aches and pains, chest pain provoked by exercise suggests an urgent heart issue; tell the doctor immediately.

Finally, work with the clinician if parkinsonism limits exercise. As discussed in Chapter 6, adequate carbidopa/levodopa therapy often allows exercise that would otherwise not be possible.

21

Hospitalization and Nursing Facilities

Keeping Everyone on the Same Page

Nearly all of us end up in the hospital for something sooner or later. The unique problems of Lewy disorders and medications can challenge hospital care teams. On a related note, some individuals with DLB or PDD may require care in a nursing facility. This may be transient, requiring rehabilitation and stabilization following a hospitalization; in other cases, it is indefinite because of the complex care necessary for DLB and PDD. In this chapter, the focus is on the care teams in these facilities. Although many staff in these settings are familiar with the medications and problems of DLB and PDD, this knowledge is not universal.

Little published literature addresses the special needs of those with PDD or DLB admitted to the hospital or living in extended care facilities. It is hoped that this chapter can be an aid in caring for those with PDD or DLB.

BACKGROUND FOR NURSES

People with DLB or PDD are, by definition, cognitively impaired. Sometimes this is associated with hallucinations or delusions. Most individuals also have dopamine deficiency states with parkinsonism. Another common component is autonomic nervous system dysfunction. This dysautonomia may be associated with bladder and bowel disorders but, more importantly, with orthostatic hypotension (potential for fainting when ambulating). Some people with PDD or DLB are mildly impaired by these problems, and others are quite compromised. What follows is a summary of crucial knowledge for nursing and paramedical staffs.

Things to Recognize about the Dementia of DLB and PDD

1. As with any dementia, novel environments are disorienting.
2. Hallucinations are a frequent component of DLB and PDD. These may be exacerbated by psychoactive medications, including narcotics for pain.
3. Carbidopa/levodopa is the least likely among the potent drugs for parkinsonism to provoke hallucinations. Other Parkinson drugs should generally not be started.
4. People with DLB or PDD commonly experience dream enactment behavior (REM sleep behavior disorder); this should not be misinterpreted as nocturnal hallucinations.
5. Anticholinergic medications for urinary urgency may cross the blood–brain barrier and impair cognition (e.g., oxybutynin). The only drug from this class that cannot get into the brain is trospium (Sanctura).

Things to Recognize about the Parkinsonism of DLB and PDD

1. Parkinsonism in this context is defined by movement problems, including at least two of four cardinal features:

slowness (bradykinesia); rigidity; tremor at rest; gait and balance disorder. These features reflect problems within the extrapyramidal (basal ganglia) system.

2. The parkinsonism of DLB and PDD primarily reflects a deficiency of brain dopamine.

3. For the parkinsonism of DLB and PDD, carbidopa/levodopa is the drug of choice; generally, other Parkinson's drugs should be avoided.

4. Carbidopa/levodopa must be taken on an empty stomach to be effective. It should be taken at least an hour before meals and at least 2 hours after the end of meals.

5. Timing of carbidopa/levodopa doses is very crucial for some patients, beyond taking it on an empty stomach. The levodopa response may be time-locked to each dose, lasting a few hours or less (this varies with the patient). Hence, adherence to scheduled carbidopa/levodopa administration is important to avoid wearing-off symptoms in certain patients.

6. Loss of the levodopa response can occur quickly, over a few minutes. The change can be dramatic, with a transition from being ambulatory to being unable to walk. This rapid change in symptoms should not be misinterpreted as psychogenic.

7. There are two formulations of carbidopa/levodopa, regular (immediate-release) and sustained-release (controlled-release) forms. These are not interchangeable, and there is no milligram-to-milligram correspondence. The regular (immediate-release) formulation is usually preferred, as it generates more predictable responses.

8. Regular (immediate-release) carbidopa/levodopa is often prescribed as the 25/100 formulation; the pill is yellow, which should make it distinguishable from other formulations. The controlled-release formulation is either dark gray, tan, or rose-colored.

9. The active ingredient of carbidopa/levodopa is levodopa, which relates to the second number in milligrams (the 100 of 25/100).

10. The first number relates to carbidopa, in milligrams. This does not penetrate into the brain but prevents nausea by blocking the premature conversion of dopamine from levodopa in the circulation.

11. There is a dose-related effect, ranging between one and three tablets of the 25/100 (immediate-release) formulation, each dose. Higher individual doses beyond three tablets do not add benefit if taken on an empty stomach.

12. Carbidopa/levodopa (immediate-release, not the controlled-release) may be crushed and mixed with applesauce if necessary, to aid administration.

13. A full dose of carbidopa/levodopa near bedtime is often necessary for sleep. It may need to be administered again during the night if the person is awake and unable to return to sleep (levodopa-off states are typically incompatible with sleep).

14. The number of carbidopa/levodopa tablets or doses per day is not of concern if the doses have been adjusted to meet the patient's needs.

Things to Recognize about Blood Pressure

1. People with DLB and PDD may be prone to orthostatic hypotension, where the blood pressure (BP) plummets to very low values when moving from sitting to standing.

2. Blood loss or diuretics may exacerbate this tendency toward orthostatic hypotension.

3. A dose of carbidopa/levodopa will tend to lower the standing BP for a few hours after each dose in susceptible people; it will revert back to normal (or even high) after that.

4. Check the standing BP before ambulating.

5. Standing systolic BP levels below 90 mmHg often translate into light-headedness and risk of fainting. This is a reasonable benchmark for determining when to worry about low standing BP levels.

6. If administering carbidopa/levodopa at bedtime or during the night, be aware of the potential for orthostatic hypotension if the patient has to walk to the bathroom.

OTHER RELATED ISSUES

Use of the Emergency Room

When is a trip to the emergency room necessary and likely to be productive? For general medical issues, such as injuries, sudden chest pain, or shortness of breath, evaluation in the emergency room is often appropriate. However, certain problems unique to DLB or PDD may be outside the usual experience of emergency room staff. These problems are often best addressed by the specialist or primary care clinician familiar with the neurologic problems. Common problems that are not easily recognized in the emergency room include the following.

- Severe anxiety or panic that occurs when the levodopa effect wears off is an occasional reason for a visit to the emergency room. As discussed in Chapter 9, this situation is best managed with another dose of carbidopa/levodopa and with strategies directed at establishing a consistent levodopa response. A more general approach is often taken by emergency staff, and a Valium-like medication is prescribed. Medications of this type include alprazolam (Xanax) and lorazepam (Ativan). While these will calm anxiety, they are sedating and may cause unsteadiness. They can indeed address the immediate problem but are not a good long-term solution.

- Faints and near-faints are common emergency room problems. However, orthostatic hypotension as the cause is rare, except in Lewy disorders. In the emergency room, recognition of orthostatic hypotension is easily missed for two reasons. First, the BP is routinely not checked in positions other than the sitting (or lying). Second, if several hours elapse from the last dose of carbidopa/levodopa, the tendency toward orthostatic hypotension may have dissipated. Recall from Chapter 13 that a dose of carbidopa/levodopa will lower the standing BP in susceptible people, beginning 30 to 60 minutes after a dose. This effect will persist for a few hours.

- Painful cramps, especially leg cramps, occur in those with Lewy disorders and are levodopa-responsive. However, this may not be recognized in the emergency room. Moreover, these cramps are sometimes incorrectly attributed to carbidopa/levodopa treatment. In fact, such cramps typically represent painful dystonias and are usually very responsive to another full dose of carbidopa/levodopa.
- Recent onset of a new confusional state occasionally has a simple explanation. If someone with DLB or PDD has been well stabilized but over a day or two becomes very disoriented or hallucinatory, superimposed medical conditions should be considered, especially new infections. A simple urinary tract infection or pneumonia might be the provocative factor. Brain scans are typically done in this setting, but usually a new brain lesion is not the cause, unless there has been a fall with head trauma.

Misconceptions

Family members occasionally encourage clinicians to admit a DLB or PDD patient into the hospital for medication adjustments. This seems sensible when the medication regimen is complicated and responses are unstable. While this was common practice more than 30 years ago, it is no longer allowed unless the problem is life-threatening, such as an extremely low blood pressure. There is no reimbursement in the United States for such medication adjustments in the hospital unless there is a life-threatening condition.

22

Families, Caregivers, and Assistance

By definition, those with DLB or PDD are cognitively impaired. The degree of cognitive impairment is highly variable; some people remain relatively compensated and stable for years. For others, confusion impairs even the simplest of activities.

Unlike Alzheimer's disease, in which dementia occurs in isolation, DLB and PDD are often associated with other problems: gait and balance dysfunction; impairment of hand dexterity; the bowel, bladder, and blood pressure problems of dysautonomia. The challenges to not only the affected person, but also the spouse or partner and family can be substantial. Caregivers may have many responsibilities, and restructured lives become the rule. These issues are so variable that a one-size-fits-all approach is not realistic.

FINANCES AND LEGAL MATTERS

Once DLB or PDD has been diagnosed, it is wise for the spouse, partner, or family to discuss with the affected patient whether revisions in decision-making should be addressed. Occasional people with DLB or PDD have relatively limited cognitive problems, and for these individuals perhaps no major changes in the family business or finances are necessary. However, this issue should still be discussed. Investments, taxes, and bill-paying may need to be switched to another family member or spouse. A family business may need new leadership. In some cases, leadership positions may be retained, but with an advisor who reviews all important decisions. When there is uncertainty, formal cognitive testing may provide important insight. Psychologists typically offer psychometric testing, assessing various aspects of cognition. The interpretation of these findings can be translated into implications for decision-making.

DRIVING

One of the most disabling restrictions placed on someone in our society is the removal of driving privileges. Communities are no longer structured where one can simply walk to the store, church, or synagogue. In the setting of DLB or PDD, however, driving restrictions or limitations may be appropriate. At least the possibility should be discussed. Driving may be compromised by both cognitive impairment and parkinsonism. Usually it is the cognitive problems that are the greater threat to the driver and public safety.

Cognitive impairment that might compromise driving safety may not be easily appreciated. People with DLB or PDD often experience difficulties with visuospatial perception, impairing their sense of three-dimensional space while driving. Also, the brain frontal lobe dysfunction, discussed in Chapter 4, may translate into poor judgment or impulsiveness, as well as poor insight.

Liability issues need to be considered in this context. Even if the driver with DLB or PDD was not at fault in an accident, a clever attorney might argue that this person should not have been driving.

The spouse, partner or family should not be put in the position of telling someone they must not drive. They may advise the person regarding driving, but imposing a driving prohibition is an untenable position for a loved one. This is an appropriate situation in which to pass the buck to the clinician. Clinicians must be willing to take the responsibility for unpopular decisions in the best interest of patients.

There are circumstances where the individual may still be a safe driver but there is no way to be sure. In this situation, a manual driving test administered by the state department of motor vehicles is an option. All states offer this service, which helps provide legal authority for continued driving if the test is passed. Even with an unrestricted driver's license, common sense should always prevail; sometimes driving on busy freeways or in crowded cities is best left for others in the family. If levodopa-off states are problematic, then driving should strictly be avoided during those times.

THE CAREGIVER

Because the clinical problems of DLB and PDD are so varied, one cannot be sure who will require a caregiver and when. When this need does surface, it is often not subtle. At that point, the spouse, partner, child, or other family member may need to become intimately involved with the care of that person. Sometimes this is on a very limited basis, with the person simply needing help with buttoning or getting in and out of the car. All too often it becomes more than a full-time job, something that demands 24-7 attention. If this is the case, there are important principles for realistically meeting these demands.

Caregiving needs to work, not just for the person with DLB or PDD, but also for the caregiver. A marriage or relationship can continue to be fulfilling long after the diagnosis, but in a fundamentally different way. The marriage vows then become especially meaningful and truly actualized. Or, for the children of someone with DLB or PDD, caregiving provides the opportunity to give back to the parent who once gave them so much. These are blessings that are hard to appreciate or acknowledge at the time because the task can be so difficult.

General Advice to Caregivers

A number of suggestions for caregivers have become apparent over the years in my clinic and are important to pass on.

- Establish an open channel of communications with the primary clinician. Be an active party to treatment. Do not be timid in speaking up or addressing true concerns.
- List the priorities that need to be addressed when visiting the clinician. The clinician needs to focus especially on the problems important to the patient and caregiver, but these may not be apparent. For example, if the clinician is focusing on medications for memory but the bigger problem is that no one is sleeping at night, voice this issue.
- Become knowledgeable about the medications. Learn the purpose of each drug and when it is best taken, and ask questions if anything is unclear. Use the knowledge imparted in this book to engage the doctor in appropriate conversation and questions. Do not be afraid to partner with the clinician in treatment.
- Become aware of physiatrists, the doctors in the departments of physical medicine and rehabilitation. The primary physician can easily request a consultation with them. This is a specialty in medicine that focuses on practical solutions to common problems of disabled patients. These clinicians are the most knowledgeable about canes, walkers, wheelchairs, and motorized scooters. They can advise about adaptations to the home that increase safety and reduce fall risk. For example, they may suggest placement of grab-bars in the bathroom or elimination of throw rugs in the hallway. Finally, they are the clinicians who direct physical therapists, who can advise and instruct in therapy, exercise, and gait programs.
- Where speech is a problem, such as a soft or garbled voice, ask the primary clinician for referral to a speech therapist. There are voice and speech therapy programs designed especially for the problems of Lewy disorders.

For the Caregiver Interacting with the More Disabled Patient

- Recognize the challenges of novelty in the setting of dementia; familiar surroundings and structured lives are often better tolerated.
- Do not underestimate the benefit of good night's sleep.
- Be one step ahead of hazards, especially fall risks. An otherwise good day is ruined by an injury in a fall.
- Hide or lock away things that might translate into trouble; this might include car keys or guns.

Maintaining Sanity While Being a 24-7 Caregiver

Becoming a caregiver can be a beautiful and loving endeavor; however, the life enrichment from caregiving needs to be complemented by other necessary life experiences. Human beings need a more diverse set of experiences to remain fresh and ready to continue. Thus, respite activities need to be an important part of the schedule. Such activities take the caregiver away from the daily responsibilities of caregiving to friendships and experiences that help break the routine.

Remember that caregiving is like a marathon, rather than a sprint. One needs to pace oneself and recognize that there is always a new day to get something done. Limits should be set so that the caregiver does not take on more than can be handled. Limits might relate to the following:

- *Heavy lifting.* Caregiving might involve true physical lifting. If the spouse or partner requires much assistance, a realistic assessment of the amount of heavy lifting and manual labor should be made. Various lifts and devices that might help are within the realm of physiatrists, who can give pertinent advice. If lifting is frequently necessary and the caregiver cannot do it, then other living arrangements may be necessary (see below).

- *Sleep deprivation.* Reversed day–night cycles, nocturnal awakening, and nighttime hallucinations may leave the caregiver devoid of adequate sleep. An occasional bad night can be tolerated, but if disruption occurs night after night, it may be impossible to continue with the caregiving. Respite from relentless night activity is necessary and may require engaging other family, hiring nighttime help, or moving the loved one to a care facility.
- *Constricted social life.* Caregiving should not terminate interactions with friends or end social events outside the home. Make time for this and do not feel guilty about finding enjoyment outside the home and away from the loved one.
- *Curtailed exercise.* Just as physical exercise was emphasized as important for those with DLB, PDD, and Parkinson's disease, it is also important for caregivers. Besides the general health benefits described in Chapters 19 and 20, a good workout is an excellent way to clear the mind and get ready for a new day.
- *Neglected health.* As a caregiver, it is easy to focus all one's attention on the health needs of the loved one. Forgetting to address one's own health does no favors to either party. Maintain an annual examination schedule with the internist or primary clinician and follow through with the recommended tests and treatments.
- *Abandoning friends.* Everyone needs someone to talk to, even when things are going well. Keep close friends apprised of activities and keep an open channel of communication. When things are not going well, use this resource to get things off the mind and provide feedback on plans.

Most importantly, learn the word *respite*. Come up for air and smell the flowers. Keep fresh by maintaining a network of friends and valued family members. Use them as a resource. Recognize when breaks are needed, including longer ones that take more than a few hours, to allow returning with renewed energy.

Use Community Resources

A variety of resources are available and may include a church or synagogue, where volunteers may welcome the opportunity to assist their neighbor in respite care. Clergy often have invaluable ideas for help. Each county should have a social service agency that can provide advice on community resources, ranging from Meals on Wheels (freeing up time that might otherwise be devoted to meal preparation) to home health care and respite care. Many communities have nursing facilities that will accept a loved one for a brief stay while the caregiver is out of town for a respite trip or a family gathering.

Matching Living Arrangements to the Needs of the Patient and Family

Many caregivers experience guilt even thinking about a residence for their loved one outside the home. However, it may not only be necessary but in the best interests of both parties. It is true that some individuals with DLB or PDD have lesser problems and are able to live in their homes indefinitely. Others, however, exceed the level of care that their family or spouse can provide. Considering better living arrangements is not a concession of weakness and need not engender guilt. Recognize the advantages for everyone, when the time is appropriate.

There is a spectrum of alternative living arrangements that may be considered, depending on the needs. Daily respite care may be sufficient for some, and adult care facilities may meet that need while the person with PDD or DLB is still residing at home. This allows the caregiver an opportunity to engage in other activities during portions of the waking day. Sometimes the home of many years is not a good fit with the current needs. Stairs may pose dangers and home maintenance may exceed capabilities. Assisted living facilities may provide an ideal situation, where a couple can still live together but with the help of staff to provide meals and respite care. Beyond this are memory-care and nursing facilities that offer a broad range of services and living opportunities for the individual with PDD or DLB. Spouses and partners will then be in a position to tend to their own needs and still visit their loved ones on a frequent basis. Love stories do not end with such separation.

Glossary

Acetylcholine—A neurotransmitter that is widely distributed in the body and brain. It is found in the autonomic nervous system and in brain memory circuits.

Alpha-synuclein—A normal molecule that is universally present in brain cells. Mutations or genetic duplications of this molecule have been identified in rare families with dominantly inherited Parkinson's disease; some members of these families developed dementia. Alpha-synuclein is present in Lewy bodies. Currently, it is suspected of playing a causative role in all Lewy disorders.

Alzheimer's disease—The most common cause of neurodegenerative dementia. Most individuals affected by this disorder have primarily cognitive symptoms. This is in contrast to dementia with Lewy bodies or Parkinson's disease with dementia, in which a variety of non-cognitive problems are present.

Autonomic nervous system—The internal set of nervous system circuits that unconsciously regulate basic functions such as digestion, bowel movements, bladder function, blood pressure, heart rate and sweating. This system is affected in Lewy disorders.

Axons—Wire-like extensions from nervous system cells (neurons) that project to other neurons to signal them.

Blood-brain-barrier—The natural barrier that restricts substances in the circulation from entering the brain.

Bradykinesia—Slowness of movement.

Bradyphrenia—Slowness of thinking.

Carbidopa—A medication that blocks dopa-decarboxylase (L-aromatic amino acid decarboxylase). Carbidopa cannot cross the blood–brain barrier and does not block dopa decarboxylase in the brain. When combined with levodopa (carbidopa/levodopa) it protects levodopa from premature conversion to dopamine in the circulation. This prevents the nausea that would otherwise be provoked by dopamine stimulating the nausea center in the brain stem where the blood–brain barrier is patent.

Cognition—The capacity to perceive, think, remember, and use language.

Cognitive—Relating to intellectual function.

COMT inhibitor—COMT stands for catechol-O-methyltransferase. This enzyme degrades levodopa. Blocking COMT with the drug entacapone (Comtan) allows levodopa to remain 30 to 60 minutes longer in the circulation.

Delusions—False beliefs in the face of incontrovertible evidence to the contrary, such as paranoid ideation or irrational convictions of spouse infidelity.

Dementia—Loss of intellectual functioning that is sufficient to impair activities of daily living. It may affect reasoning, judgment, perception, or memory. If treatable causes have been ruled out, this typically represents a neurodegenerative condition.

Dementia with Lewy bodies (DLB)—The second most common cause of neurodegenerative dementia. In this disorder, the cognitive impairment is associated with other problems, including parkinsonism as well as impaired autonomic system function. Lewy bodies are found under the microscope in affected brain regions.

Dendrites—Nervous system cells (neurons) communicate with one another by releasing a tiny amount of a specific brain chemical (neurotransmitter), which activates the next neuron. Neurons have wire-like extensions for receiving these signals, called dendrites.

Dopamine—A neurotransmitter that is lost in Parkinson's disease and in dementia with Lewy bodies, due to degeneration of the nigrostriatal neurons in the brain.

Dopamine agonist—A class of drugs used to treat Parkinson's disease. These medications act like synthetic forms of dopamine, directly stimulating dopamine receptors.

Functional MRI—Brain MRI done before and after specific simple tasks that allows computer computation to document brain regions activated by the task. For example, if the task is mental arithmetic, the brain regions used to do mental arithmetic can be imaged.

Hallucination—Implies seeing illusory images or hearing voices that are not real. In Lewy disorders, visual hallucinations are the rule, whereas hearing voices is very uncommon.

Levodopa (L-dopa)—A natural amino acid that is the precursor to the neurotransmitter dopamine. It is the most efficacious medication for treatment of Parkinson's disease. In the present era, it is administered with carbidopa (carbidopa/levodopa), which protects it from premature metabolism.

Lewy body—A collection of material within neurons that is seen under the microscope through use of special stains. Smaller collections may be found within the processes of neurons, termed Lewy neurites. This is the biological hallmark of Parkinson's disease as well as dementia with Lewy bodies.

Lewy neurodegeneration—Disease of nervous system circuits marked by the presence of Lewy bodies and Lewy neurites seen under the microscope.

MAO-B inhibitor—MAO stands for monoamine oxidase. This enzyme is present inside and outside the brain. There are two forms of MAO, A and B. The B-form (MAO-B) can typically be blocked safely, and the primary drugs for that purpose are rasagiline (Azilect) and selegiline. If MAO-A is blocked by other drugs, then a special diet and avoidance of numerous medications is mandated.

Mild cognitive impairment (MCI)—Impaired thinking, memory, or judgment (cognition) that is not so severe as to substantially interfere with activities of daily living.

Motor—Synonymous with movement. Brain *motor* control circuits control the movement of limbs, body, and face as well as speech.

MRI scan—Magnetic resonance imaging scanning can be performed on any region of the body and is especially useful for study of the brain.

Neurodegeneration—The demise (degeneration) of specific brain cells, suggesting a premature death or aging. Neurodegenerative diseases encompass many conditions, such as Alzheimer's disease, Parkinson's disease, and Lou Gehrig's disease (amyotrophic lateral sclerosis). These are all independent from one another and are each marked by susceptibility of specific neuronal systems, sparing other brain regions.

Neurotransmitter—A nervous system molecule that is released at the end of the neuron to signal the next neuron in the brain circuit.

Neuron—The fundamental cell of the nervous system. It has a cell body, similar to other cells. However, it also has a long wire-like extension, the axon, for transmitting signals to other cells. Other wire-like extensions of the cell body, called dendrites, receive the signals from other neurons.

Neurotransmitter—The signaling chemical released by neurons to activate or inhibit the activity of another neuron.

Nigrostriatal—The pathway from the substantia nigra to the striatum. This is traversed by neurons having a cell body in the substantia nigra, with the axon projecting to the striatum. The neurotransmitter is dopamine.

Orthostatic hypotension—A substantial drop in blood pressure when going from sitting or lying to standing. It may be sufficient to result in faintness or actual fainting.

Parkinsonism—A condition having the features of Parkinson's disease. Parkinsonism is defined as having at least two of the following cardinal features: slowness (bradykinesia), stiffness (rigidity), tremor at rest, and gait or balance problems. Thus, any disorder that looks like Parkinson's disease may be termed parkinsonism, even if it has another cause.

Parkinson's disease (PD)—A Lewy body neurodegenerative disorder with clinical features of parkinsonism (see above) and typically responsive to levodopa treatment, reflecting brain dopamine deficiency. With progression, the parkinsonism may become incompletely responsive to levodopa treatment, plus dementia and dysautonomia may develop.

Parkinson's disease with dementia (PDD)—Parkinson's disease that has progressed and subsequently affected cognition. Under the microscope it is essentially identical to dementia with Lewy bodies (DLB). If parkinsonism occurs first and the dementia starts more than a year later it is called Parkinson's disease with dementia (PDD). If the parkinsonism and dementia start within a year of each other, it is termed dementia with Lewy bodies. This is an arbitrary definition established by a consensus panel.

Pseudobulbar affect—A neurologic symptom that manifests as crying or laughing in response to stimuli that are only mildly emotion-provoking. Those affected by pseudobulbar crying note that they typically will not feel particularly sad but nonetheless cry uncontrollably. Pseudobulbar laughter is less frequent.

SSRI—Stands for selective serotonin reuptake inhibitor, which is an antidepressant medication class that includes Prozac (fluoxetine) and many related drugs. They all facilitate the neurotransmission of brain serotonin. This neurotransmitter is thought to be important for a sense of well-being, and low serotonin activity has been related to psychological depression.

Synapse—The interface of one neuronal process with a second neuron. At this interface, the terminal end of the axon releases a neurotransmitter that activates a specific receptor on the next neuron in that circuit. The submicroscopic space between that terminal and receptor is the synapse.

Terminals—Nervous system cells (neurons) send out long extensions (axons) that terminate as an out-pouching region, called the terminal. This is where the neurotransmitter is stored, to be released at the synapse.

Index

Page numbers followed by an italicized *t* indicate a table. Page numbers in *italics* indicate a figure.

A

abdominal binder, 155–156
Abilify (aripiprazole), 102
Accupril (quinapril), 151
ACE-inhibitors, 151
acetylcholine (neurotransmitter), 57, 130–131, 133, 158, 169, 245
acetylcholine blocking agents (anticholinergics), 57
acetylcholinesterase inhibitors, 130–134. *see also* donepezil; galantamine; rivastigmine
Actonel (risedronate), 209
Adalat (nifedipine), 151
Advil PM (ibuprofen and diphenhydramine), 181
Advisory Panel (U.S. FDA), 20
aerobic exercise, 22–23, 221–222, 227
aggression/acting out behaviors, 136–138
akathisia (inner restlessness), 97, 106, 135
Aldactone (spironolactone), 152
alendronate (Fosamax), 209
alertness fluctuations, in DLB and PDD, 35
alfuzosin (Uroxatral), 167
alpha-blockers
   for prostate enlargement, 152, 167
   side effects, in orthostatic hypotension, 152
alpha-synuclein genetic coding, 16–17
alpha-synuclein protein
   Braak's background work, 8, 17–18
   discovery/background, 16–17
   identification of, 6
   multiple system atrophy and, 193–194
   toxicity transformation process, 17
alprazolam (Xanax), 102, 127*t*, 137, 189*t*, 235

Altace (ramipril), 151
Alzheimer's disease, 3, 6, 7
   DLB comparison with, 12, 31–32, 34
   isolated dementia in, 237
   memantine treatment in, 134–135
   microscopic hallmarks, 12
   PDD comparison with, 31–32, 34
amantadine, 57–58, 68, 86
Ambien (zolpidem), 185
amiloride (Midamor), 152
amitriptyline (Elavil), 127*t*, 153, 178, 182, 190, 200, 203
amlodipine (Norvasc), 151
amyotrophic lateral sclerosis (ALS), 3
Angiotensin II-receptor blockers, 151
anticholinergics
   as bad choice, in DLB and PDD, 57
   elimination of, for those already on medications
      benztropine (Cogentin), 82–83
      trihexyphenidyl (Artane), 82–83, 112
   hallucinations caused by, 112
   information for nurses, 232
   mechanism of action, 133–134
   side effects, 232
antidepressant drugs. *see also* selective serotonin reuptake inhibitors; tricyclic antidepressants
   for behavioral problems, 137–138
   contraindicated combinations, 205–206
   low dose, as sleep aid, 182
   in non-disabling depression, 203–205
   in nonsuicidal, prominent depression, 201–203
   possible side effects, 153, 178, 194
antihistamines, 181

antihypertensive medications, 150–151
anti-nausea medications, 58–59, 74
antipsychotics (neuroleptics), 59, 102–103, 182. *see also* aripiprazole; haloperidol; olanzapine; risperidone; ziprasidone
anxiety, in DLB and PDD, 39, 53
  carbidopa/levodopa treatment
    anxiety/panic coming and going, 103–104
    anxiety present continuously, 103
  quetiapine drug class, 104–105
  treatment alternatives
    antipsychotics (neuroleptics), 102–103
    benzodiazepines, 104
    ECT therapy, 105
    environmental strategies, 105
    Prozac class of drugs, 105
    quetiapine drug class, 104
    typical/atypical neuroleptics, 104–105
apathy, in DLB and PDD, 40
apomorphine (dopamine agonist), 10
Aricept (donepezil), 113, 115, 131–132
aripiprazole (Abilify), 102
armodafinil (Nuvigil), 178, 191–192
Artane (trihexyphenidyl), 57
Atacand (candesartan), 151
Atelvia (risedronate), 209
atenolol (Tenormin), 151
Ativan (lorazepam), 102
automatic movement difficulties, 37
autonomic nervous system
  blood pressure control by, 18, 25, 29–31, 139, 214, 245
  described, *29,* 29–30, 139
  Lewy neurodegenerative influences
    bladder problems, 11, 12, 43, 139
    constipation, 11–12, 37, 43, 139
    dysautonomia, 37–38
    orthostatic hypotension, 11, 43, 75–77, 139
  link with central nervous system, 139
Avapro (irbesartan), 151
Avodart (dutasteride), 167
Azilect (rasagiline), 55, 56, 68, 85

B
balance/imbalance issues
  as medication side effect, 102, 104, 185, 196
  as symptom, 37, 52, 54, 148, 210, 233
basal ganglia regions (brain)
  apathy and, 40
  body movement modulation by, 28
  components of, 26, *27*

degeneration in parkinsonism of DLB, PDD, 28, 37, 233
  improper functioning in parkinsonism, 49
benazepril (Lotensin), 151
benserazide/levodopa, 55, 78–79
benzodiazepines
  management considerations, 102
  possible side effects, 104, 112, 127*t,* 137, 189*t,* 196
benztropine (Cogentin), 57, 68, 82–83
beta-blockers, 151
bisphosphonate drugs, 209
bladder
  autonomic regulation of, 18, 25, 29–31, *30*
  description, 162, *162*
  men/women, aging issues, 163
  nighttime urination, 184–185
  related DLB, PDD conditions
    control difficulties, 43–44
    neurogenic bladder, 161, 163, 165–166
    prostate gland involvement, 161, 163, 165–167
    treatments, 127*t,* 133–134, 164–167
    urge incontinence, 164–165
    urinary hesitancy, 161, 163, 165–166
    urinary tract infections, 113, 115, 128, 163–167, 236
Blocadren (timolol), 151
blood-brain barrier, 10
blood pressure (BP). *see also* orthostatic hypotension
  autonomic control of, 18, 25, 29–31, 139, 214, 245
  drugs for raising
    extra carbidopa, 156
    fludrocortisone, 156
    midodrine, 156–158
    pyridostigmine, 158
  drugs that cause lowering, 167
  exercise recommendation, 228
  information for nurses, 234–235
  leukoaraiosis and, 214
  lowering, if high when reclining, 158–159
  measurement, values of concern, 144–145
  normal values, 75, 142–143
  salt intake/restriction recommendation, 210
  sleep apnea influences on, 187
  things to recognize about, 234–235
Boniva (ibandronate), 209

bowels
autonomic regulation of, 18, 25, 29, *29,*
31, 139
constipation problems, 11, 12, 43, 139
chronic, with impaction, 172–173
drug-related exacerbation of, 169–170
measures for non-response, 171–172
treatment, 170–171
irritable bowel syndrome, treatment, 127*t*
Braak, Heikko, 8, 17–18
bradykinesia
as classic Parkinson's symptom, 9
defined, 36, 49–50
manifestations of, 50
brain. *see also* basal ganglia regions; cortex;
substantia nigra
arterial atherosclerosis, 7
brain stem/substantia nigra, *28*
central nervous system connections, *26*
CT/MRI diagnostic scans, 41–42
exercise influences on, 223–224, 225–226
Lewy degeneration in, 8–9
nucleus basalis, *130,* 131–132
primary cortices (lobes), *32*
spinal cord interface with, 25–29, *26–28*
vascular health and osteoporosis, 214
brain imaging, 4, 41–42, 128, 222–223.
see also computed tomography;
magnetic resonance imaging
brain neuroplasticity, 23
brain volume, exercise influences on,
223–224

C
Calan (verapamil), 151
calcium-channel blockers, 151
candesartan (Atacand), 151
Capgras syndrome, 40, 111
Capoten (captopril), 151
captopril (Capoten), 151
carbidopa
anti-nausea properties, 55
benserazide similarity, 64
levodopa without, 63
mechanism of action, 63–64
properties of, 63
carbidopa/levodopa. *see also* carbidopa/
levodopa, forms; carbidopa/
levodopa, side effects; carbidopa/
levodopa, treatment principles
alternative medication choices, 56–57
anxiety reduction from, 39
benserazide comparison, 78–79

blood pressure influences of, 234–235
dopamine agonist comparison, 56
entacapone use with, 55, 56, 87
life span improvement from, 21–22
long-duration response, 89–90
mechanisms of action, 45, 62–64, 68
for non-motor parkinsonism symptoms,
61
for parkinsonism symptoms, 10, 23, 36,
42, 47
as primary treatment of parkinsonism in
DLB, PDD, 58
short-duration response, 90–91
treatment choice decisions, 56
types of/dosage information for nurses,
233–234
without carbidopa, 63
carbidopa/levodopa, forms. *See also* Sinemet
in combinations
side effects, 81–82
dosages, extended vs. immediate release,
65–66
extended-release, 64–65
regular, immediate-release
dosage escalation, 69–70
pill sizes, 66–67
reasons for choosing, 64–65
treatment initiation, 72*b*
Stalevo usage, 55, 56, 67
without carbidopa, 63
carbidopa/levodopa, side effects
akathisia, 97, 106, 135
in combinations, 81–82
dyskinesias, 95–96
dystonia, 96–97
hallucinations, 77–78
nausea, 73–74
orthostatic hypotension, 75–77, 76–77, 95,
145–146
short-duration pattern, 94–95
tremor, 97
carbidopa/levodopa, treatment principles,
68–73
actions for lack of benefits,
72–73
in anxiety, in DLB and PDD
coming and going, 103–104
continuously present, 103
dosage regulation
at bedtime/during the night,
94
for comes and goes parkinsonism, 93
escalation, 69–70

carbidopa/levodopa (*Cont.*)
  dosage regulation (*Cont.*)
    in insomnia, in DLB and PDD, 106–107
    for poorly controlled all day long
        parkinsonism, 92–93
    relation to meals, 68–69
    tablets for day concerns, 93
  initiation of treatment, 71, 72*b*
  in pain, 107–108
  targeting of symptoms, 70–71
Cardene (nicardipine), 151
Cardizem (diltiazem), 151
Cardura (doxazosin), 152, 167
caregivers
  attention required of, 239
  general advice for, 240
  interacting with disabled patient, 241
  maintaining sanity/limit setting by,
      241–242
  respite needs of, 242
carvedilol (Coreg), 152
catechol-*O*-methyl-transferase (COMT)
      inhibitors, 55, 86–87. *see also*
      entacapone; Stalevo; tolcapone
central nervous system
  brain/basal ganglia regions, 27
  brain connections, 26
  brain stem/substantia nigra, 28
  Lewy body location, 18
  link with autonomic nervous system, 139
  organization, cortex to spinal cord,
      23–29
  prototypic neuron, 27
cerebrospinal fluid (CSF) examination,
      128–129
cerebrovascular disease, 7
chlorthalidone, 152
cholesterol elevation, 7
clinical trials
  aerobic exercise, 221–222, 227
  coenzyme Q10, 21
  pramipexole, 19, 56, 77–78
  rasagiline, 20
  ropinirole, 19, 56, 77–78
  rotigotine, 56
  Rytary, 65
  selegiline (deprenyl), 19
  vitamin E, 19
  vitamins B6, B12, 212
clonazepam (Klonopin), 102, 127*t*, 189*t*,
      190, 196
clozapine (Clozaril), 59, 103, 113–114,
      189–190

coenzyme Q_{10}, 20–21, 213
Cogentin (benztropine), 57
Cognex (tacrine), 131
cognition. *see also* dementia
  defined, 5, 123
  exercise benefits, 22–23, 222
  impairment from medication, 102, 127*t*
  Lewy body neurodegeneration and, 9, 31
  medication for
    acetylcholinesterase inhibitors, 130–134
    dopamine, 135
    NMDA inhibitor, 134–135
  mental clarity fluctuations, 126
  non-drug treatment strategies, 135
  possible restrictions in, 136
  profile of DLB, PDD, 12, 31–35
    delusions, 35
    executive function, 32–33
    hallucinations, 35
    memory, 34–35
    thinking/alertness fluctuations, 35
    visuospatial function, 33–34
  psychometric assessment of, 41
  symptoms in PDD, 11
community resources, 243
Compazine (prochlorperazine), 58, 74
compressive hose, 154–155
compulsive behaviors, caused by dopamine
      agonists. *see* gambling behaviors;
      spending behaviors
computed tomography (CT) brain scan,
      41, 128
Comtan (entacapone), 55–56, 62, 67, 86–87,
      246
Concerta (methylphenidate), 179, 191–192
constipation problems
  anticholinergic exacerbation, 82–83,
      169–170
  autonomic involvement, 11–12, 37, 43,
      139
  chronic, with impaction, 172–173
  drug-related exacerbation of,
      169–170
  medication exacerbation
    anticholinergics, 82–83, 169–170
    trospium, 185
  treatment, 170–171
    measures for non-response, 171–172
Coreg (carvedilol), 152
Corgard (nadolol), 151
cortex (brain), 8, 8–9, 26
  description, 31
  executive skill mediation role, 32

Lewy degeneration in, *8,* 8–9
spinal cord connections with, 26, *26,* 28
visuospatial perception, conception role,
34
Cozaar (losartan), 151
cramp-like contractions, 108
creatine, 20
cyclobenzaprine, 127*t*

D
Dalmane (flurazepam), 190
daytime drowsiness. *see also* sleep disorders
causes of, 38–39, 177–178
drug treatment, 178–179, 191–192
fluctuating nature of, 35
hallucinations and, 113
impaired thinking from, 129
from medications, 189–190, 189*t*
signs of, 177
Daytrana (methylphenidate), 179, 191–192
delusions
in Capgras syndrome, 111
defined, 35, 40, 111, 246
in DLB and PDD, 35, 39, 40, 42
as medication side effect, 56–57, 81–83,
85, 112–113, 121, 191–192, 205
medication treatment for, 59, 113–115,
134, 137, 182, 189
Demadex (torsemide), 152
dementia, 125–138. *see also* dementia with
Lewy bodies; Parkinson's disease with
dementia
aggression/acting out behaviors, 136–138
assessment tools, 4
cognition medications, 130–135
defined, 4, 125
in isolation, in Alzheimer's, 237
search for treatable causes
blood work, urinalysis, 128
brain scan assessment, 128
medication list, 127*t*
psychometrics assessment, 129–130
sleep disorder treatment, 129
spinal fluid examination, 128–129
spectrum in Lewy body conditions, ix
dementia with Lewy bodies (DLB). *see also*
depression, in DLB and PDD
Alzheimer brain pathology in, 7
Alzheimer's disease comparison, 4, 12
brain aging contribution to, 7
causative for neurodegenerative dementia,
4, 6, 11–12, 28
cognitive profile, 31–35

delusions, 35
executive function, 32–33
hallucinations, 35
memory, 34–35
thinking/alertness fluctuations, 35
visuospatial function, 33–34
contributing factors, 6–7
diagnosis, 40–43
diagnostic difficulties, 15
dopamine deficiencies in, 10, 47
dysautonomia in, 37–38
excessive sleep component, 190–191
hallmarks of, 5
hospitalization/background for nurses,
232
levodopa treatment, 47
name derivation, 13
nucleus basalis degeneration in, *130,*
131–132
parkinsonism of, 36–37
hospitalization/background for nurses,
232–234
Parkinson's symptoms in, 10, 12
PDD distinctions from, 13
pharmacologic treatment guidelines,
55–57
psychiatric symptoms in, 39–40
sleep disorders in, 38–39
symptom mechanisms, 18
thinking/memory problems in, x
treatment guidelines, 55–57
depression, in DLB and PDD, 39, 53, 135
apathy caused by, 40
assessment, 129
of severity, 200–201
of true depression, 199–200
cognition influenced by, 135
from medication withdrawal, 83, 122,
191–192
physiological basis of, 39
treatment, non-pharmacologic
for dark thoughts, suicidal ideation, 201
depression, non-suicidal, 201–203
electroconvulsive therapy, 206
non-disabling depression, 203–205
treatment, pharmacologic
parkinsonism and SSRIs, 206
selegiline-rasagiline interactions,
205–206
side effects of, 178
SSRIs, 105, 112, 200
tricyclic drugs, 127*t,* 169–170, 200
variance of intensity, 11

desipramine (Norpramine), 153, 203
diabetes mellitus, 7
diagnosis
  of DLB, 12, 40–43
    brain imaging, 41
    diagnostic criteria, 42–43
    history, 41
    neurological examination, 41
  of Parkinson's disease, 6
  of PDD, 43
diazepam (Valium), 102, 127*t*, 189*t*, 190
diltiazem (Cardizem, Tiazac, Dilacor), 151
Diovan (valsartan), 151
diphenhydramine, 181
disturbed sleep architecture, 39
diuretics (water pills), 147, 152, 164, 184, 234
dizziness
  defined, 148
  in low blood pressure, 77, 148, 154
  as medication side effect, 134
  vestibular (inner ear) dizziness, 148–149
domperidone, 58–59, 74
donepezil (Aricept), 113, 115, 131–132
dopamine (brain dopamine), 9–10
  carbidopa/levodopa's influence on, 45
  cognition and, 135
  deficiencies in DLB, PDD, 10, 28–29
  information for nurses, 233
  insomnia and, 38
  levodopa as precursor to, 10, 47
  need for, for movement, 47
  pill form limitations, 47
  substantia nigra use of, 28
dopamine agonists, 10, 19, 55. *see also*
    apomorphine; pramipexole;
    ropinirole; rotigotine
  elimination, for those taking medications
    pramipexole, extended release, 84
    pramipexole, regular release, 83–84
    ropinirole, extended release, 84
    ropinirole, regular-release, 84
    rotigotine patch, 84–85
  pathological behaviors provoked by,
      117–120
    drug tapering treatment, 121–122
    mechanisms of action, 120
    recognition of behaviors, 119
    risk factors, 120
dopamine blocking drugs. *see also*
    metoclopramide; prochlorperazine
  for nausea, 58–59
  for psychosis, 59
dopamine replacement medication

drug choice
  COMT inhibitors, 55
  dopamine agonists, 10, 19, 55
  levodopa, 54–55
  MAO-B inhibitors, 19–20, 55
  levodopa comparison, 56
  treatment determination criteria, 53–54
doxazosin (Cardura), 152, 167
doxepin (Sinequan), 127*t*, 153, 182, 190, 203
dream enactment behavior. *see* REM sleep
      behavior disorder
driving restrictions, dealing with, 238–239
dutasteride (Avodart), 167
Dyazide (triamterene), 152
DynaCirc (isradipine), 151
dysautonomia in PDD and DLB, 37–38, 75
dyskinesias
  amantadine treatment, 58, 62, 86, 98–99
  causes, 95
  defined, 95
  as levodopa side effect, 94, 95–96
  reduction strategy, 86
  treatment strategy, 96
dystonia
  defined, 96
  examples of, 96–97
  treatment, 97
  types of, 108

E
eating compulsivity, from dopamine
      agonists, 57, 118–119
eating/meals
  and carbidopa/levodopa administration,
      68–69
  falling asleep during, 177
  orthostatic hypotension exacerbation
      from, 146–147
  utensils and tremors, 53
  vitamin supplementation and, 211
Elavil (amitriptyline), 127*t*, 153, 178, 182,
      190, 200, 203
Eldepryl (selegiline), 55, 62, 68
electroconvulsive therapy (ECT)
  for depression, 206
  for prominent anxiety, 105
emergency room
  uses of, 235–236
  visits with patients, 102, 190
enalapril (Vasotec), 151
entacapone (Comtan), 62, 67, 86–87, 246
  levodopa with, 55, 56, 87
erectile dysfunction drugs (for males), 152

essential tremor, 36, 53, 151
eszopiclone (Lunesta), 185
Evista (raloxifene), 209
executive function
    frontal cortex role in, 32
    profile of DLB, PDD, 32–33, 125
Exelon patch (rivastigmine), 113
exercise
    aerobic, clinical trials, 221–222, 227
    animal studies, 224–225
    benefits, evidence of, 219–224
    brain changes from, 223–224, 225–226
    choice of routine, 219
    cognition, benefits for, 22–23, 222
    diabetics, benefits for, 228
    osteoporosis, benefits for, 209, 215, 228
    types of, 226–228
    vigorous exercise treatment, 218–219

F
faintness, in orthostatic hypotension, 11, 37,
        75–77, 143–145, 148–150, 249
falls/falling. *see also* balance/imbalance
        issues; dizziness
    confused mental state and, 236
    osteoporosis and, 207–208
    out of bed, 195–196
    reducing risk factors, 240–241
    risk factors, 102, 182, 196, 207–208
families/partners of DLB, PDD patients
    aid for patient in mild dementia, 125
    alliance with clinicians, xi, 4, 119, 136
    community resources, 243
    depression of, 199
    driving restrictions, dealing with, 238–239
    emergency room visits with patients, 102,
        190
    financial/legal concerns, 237–238
    matching needs-based living
        arrangements, 243–244
    need for medication awareness, 196
    possible caregiving role of, 239–242
    recognition of changed behavior by, 33, 119
Farrer, Matthew, 16
felodipine (Plendil), 151
finasteride (Proscan), 167
5-alpha-reductase inhibitors, 167
Flomax (tamsulosin), 167
Florinef (fludrocortisone), 156
fludrocortisone (Florinef), 156
flurazepam (Dalmane), 190
food. *see* eating/meals
Forteo (teriparatide), 209

Fosamax (alendronate), 209
furosemide (Lasix), 152

G
gait problems, x–xi, 10, 37, 51, 90, 210, 220,
        233. *see also* balance/imbalance
        issues; falls/falling; walking
        difficulties
galantamine (Razadyne), 131, 133–134
gambling behaviors, from dopamine
        agonists, 58, 83, 109, 117–118
Geodon (ziprasidone), 102
glutamate (neurotransmitter), 98, 134
Golbe, Lawrence, 16

H
Haldol (haloperidol), 102
hallucinations
    causes of, 112–113
    commonness of, 111–112
    in DLB and PDD, 35, 40
    information for nurses, 232
    as medication side effect, 55–56, 67,
        112–113
        amantadine, 58, 86, 98
        anticholinergics, 112
        benzodiazepines, 112
        carbidopa/levodopa combinations, 112
        dopamine agonists, 112
        management, 77–78
        MAO-B inhibitors, 85
        muscle relaxants, 112
        prescription pain medications, 112
        Valium class drugs, 112
    medication treatment
        clozapine, 113–114
        donepezil, 113
        quetiapine, 113–115
        rivastigmine, 113
haloperidol (Haldol), 59, 102
HCTZ (hydrochlorothiazide), 152
hospitalization, for DLB, PDD
    background for nurses
        about blood pressure, 234–235
        about dementia of DLB, and PDD, 232
        about parkinsonism of DLB, PDD,
            232–234
    emergency room use, 235–236
    misconceptions, 236
hydrochlorothiazide (HCTZ), 152
hydrocodone, 112, 127*t*, 189*t*
hypersexual behavior, from dopamine
        agonists, 118, 119

hypertension. *see* blood pressure
hypokinetic dysarthria, 53
hypophonia, 53
Hytrin (terazosin), 152, 167

I
ibandronate (Boniva), 209
imbalance. *see* balance/imbalance issues
imipramine (Tofranil), 153
immediate-release levodopa
  dosage escalation, 69–70
  pill sizes, 66–67
  reasons for choosing, 64–65
  treatment initiation, 72*b*
indapamide (Lozol), 152
Inderal (propranolol), 151
insomnia, x, 38, 53
  carbidopa/levodopa
    dosages, 106
    Sinemet CR vs. regular, 107
    timing of dosage, 106–107
  daytime drowsiness caused by, 177–178
  hallucinations from, 113
  Prozac class drugs causative for, 178
  RLS causative for, 179
irbesartan (Avapro), 151
irritable bowel syndrome, drugs for, 127*t*
Isoptin (verapamil), 151
isradipine (DynaCirc), 151

K
kicking movements, 26
Klonopin (clonazepam), 102, 127*t*, 189*t*,
  190, 196

L
Lasix (furosemide), 152
leukoaraiosis, 7, 214
levodopa-induced dyskinesias, 95–96
Lewy ("at rest") tremor, 10, 36, 52
Lewy bodies
  defined, x, 5, 5–6
  preparation for viewing, 6
  severity spectrum, xii
Lewy neurites, 17
Lewy tremor, 52
lightheadedness
  case example, 141
  in orthostatic hypotension, 77, 141,
    143–145, 149
lisinopril (Prinivil, Zestril), 151
Lodosyn (carbidopa), 74, 156
Lopressor (metoprolol), 151

lorazepam (Ativan), 102, 127*t*
losartan (Cozaar), 151
Lotensin (benazepril), 151
Lou Gehrig disease (amyotrophic lateral
    sclerosis), 3
Lozol (indapamide), 152
Lunesta (eszopiclone), 185

M
Madopar (benserazide and levodopa), 78–79
magnetic resonance imaging (MRI), of the
    brain
  atherosclerosis of small arteries, 7, 214
  brain tumors, 128
  brain volume, 223
  cognitive deficit assessment f, 41
  defined, 248
  exercise benefits, 222–223
Mayo Jacksonville, 16
McKeith, Ian, 42–43
McKeith diagnostic criteria, 42–43
melatonin, 181, 196
memantine (Namenda), 98–99, 134–135
Mestinon (pyridostigmine), 158
methylphenidate (Concerta), 178, 191–192
methylphenidate, extended-release
    (Concerta), 179
metoclopramide (Reglan), 58, 74
metoprolol (Lopressor, Toprol), 151
Micardis (telmisartan), 151
Midamor (amiloride), 152
midodrine (ProAmatine), 156–158
mild cognitive impairment (MCI), 4–5, 28,
    125, 222, 248
Mini-Mental State Examination, 4
minocycline, 20
Mirapex (pramipexole), 55
  extended-release (ER), 84
  possible side effects, 56, 112, 118, 190
  regular-release, 83
  in restless legs syndrome, 117, 179
  sleepiness induced by, 190
  slow elimination consideration, 62
mirtazapine (Remeron), 153
modafinil (Provigil), 178, 191–192
monoamine oxidase B (MAO-B) inhibitors,
    19–20, 55, 56, 205–206. *see also*
    rasagiline; selegiline
movement. *see also* bradykinesia; gait
    problems; rigidity (stiffness)
  automatic movement difficulties, 37,
    50–51
  basal ganglia control of, 28

classic parkinsonism symptoms, 36, 47
  impaired repetitive movements, 50
  periodic leg movements of sleep, 39
  role of dopamine for, 47
MRI (magnetic resonance imaging)
  brain scans, 7
multiple system atrophy (MSA), 193–194
muscle relaxants, 127*t*

N
nadolol (Corgard), 151
Namenda (memantine), 98–99, 134–135
narcotic pain medications, 112, 127*t*
National Institute of Health, 21
nausea
  levodopa without carbidopa as cause of,
    63
  medications for reducing
    carbidopa, 55, 66–67, 74
    dopamine blockers, 58–59
  as medication side effect, 58–59, 73–74
Neupro patch (rotigotine), 55, 62, 83, 84–85,
    112, 117. *see also* rotigotine
neurogenic bladder
  defined, 161
  urinary hesitancy from, 163, 166
  treatment, 165
neuron (prototypic), *27*
neurotransmitters. *see also*
        acetylcholinesterase inhibitors;
        dopamine
  acetylcholine, 57, 130–131, 133, 158, 169,
    245
  amantadine interaction with, 98
  defined, 9–10, 45, 248
  drugs for targeting, in parkinsonism,
    57–58
  glutamate, 98, 134
  mechanics of release, *27*, 27–28
  norepinephrine, 39, 202
  role in depression, 39
  role in Parkinson's disease, 47
  serotonin, 201–202
nicardipine (Cardene), 151
nifedipine (Adalat, Procardia), 151
NMDA (glutamate) inhibitor. *see* memantine
non-motor symptoms, of parkinsonism,
    53, 61
norepinephrine (neurotransmitter), 39, 202
Norpramin (desipramine), 153, 203
nortriptyline (Pamelor), 127*t*, 153, 200
Norvasc (amlodipine), 151
nurses, background information for

about blood pressure, in DLB, PDD,
    234–235
  about dementia of DLB, PDD, 232
  about parkinsonism of DLB, PDD,
    232
Nuvigil (armodafinil), 178, 191–192

O
olanzapine (Zyprexa), 102
ondansetron (Zofran), 58, 74
orthostatic hypotension
  carbidopa/levodopa-induced, 76–77, 95,
    145–146
  commonness in DLB, PDD, 30
  defined, 37, 75, 141–142
  dizziness in, 77, 148, 154
  eating exacerbation of, 146–147
  faintness in, 11, 37, 75–77, 143–145,
    148–150, 249
  lightheadedness in, 77, 141, 143–145,
    149
  medications causative for
    ACE-inhibitors, 151
    alpha-blockers, 152
    Angiotensin II-receptor blockers, 151
    antidepressants, 153
    antihypertensives, 150–151
    beta-blockers, 151
    calcium-channel blockers,
      151
    carbidopa/levodopa, 76–77, 95,
      145–146, 147
    carvedilol (Coreg), 152
    diuretics, 152
    male erectile dysfunction drugs,
      152
  normal blood pressure values, 75,
    142–143
  risk factors in DLB, PDD, 143
  self-assessment of, 145
  in sitting position, 153
  sudden faintness vs., 149
  systolic BP benchmarks, 144
  treatment, drug alternatives,
    153–156
    abdominal binder, 155–156
    compressive hose, 154–155
  treatment, pharmacological
    extra carbidopa, 74, 156
    fludrocortisone, 156
    midodrine, 156–158
    pyridostigmine, 158
osteopenia, 208

osteoporosis
  assessment/DEXA scan, 207–208, 209
  bisphosphonate drugs, 209
  causes, 208
  description, 207
  falls and, 207–208
  treatment
    calcium, 208, 211
    carbidopa/levodopa with vitamins,
      211–213
    coenzyme Q_{10}, 20–21, 213
    copper, 211
    dietary suggestions, 210
    exercise, 209, 215, 228
    hormone drugs, 209
    vitamin B12, 211
    vitamin D, 208–209, 210–211
oxycodone, 112, 127*t*, 189*t*

P
pain medications, narcotic and nonnarcotic,
  112, 127*t*
pain treatment, in DLB and PDD, 107–108
Pamelor (nortriptyline), 127*t*, 153
paranoia, 40, 56
parkinsonism
  animal studies of exercise, 224–225
  automatic movement difficulties in, 37,
    50–51
  bradykinesia in, 9, 36, 49–50
  cause of, 49
  classic movement symptoms, 36, 47
  defined, 29
  of DLB, and PDD, 36–37
    hospitalization/background for nurses,
      232–234
  drugs for, 127*t*
  gait problems in, x–xi, 10, 36, 51
  hypophonia/hypokinetic dysarthria in, 53
  imbalance problems in, 37, 52
  impaired repetitive movements in, 50
  in Lewy conditions, xi, 12
  non-movement symptoms, 53
  possible absence in DLB, 13, 18
  rigidity in, 10, 36, 51
  SSRI drugs and, 206
  stooped posture in, 37, 52
Parkinson's disease
  Braak's background work, 8, 17–18
  carbidopa/levodopa treatment, 45
  causes, 15
  description, 3, 8–9
  Lewy body as brain-marker of, x, 5–6, 8

  substantia nigra degeneration in, 28
  symptomatic treatment, 10
  symptoms, 9, 10–11
  treatment options, 19–23
    aerobic exercise, 22–23
    carbidopa/levodopa, 45
    coenzyme Q10, 20–21
    creatine, 20
    dopamine agonists, 19
    experimental agents, 19–20
    levodopa, 21–22
    minocycline, 20
    monoamine oxidase B inhibitors, 19–20
    vitamin E, 19
Parkinson's disease with dementia (PDD).
    see also depression, in DLB and PDD
  Alzheimer brain pathology in, 7
  brain aging contribution to, 7
  causative for dementia, 4, 6
  cognitive profile, 11, 31–35
    delusions, 35
    executive function, 32–33
    hallucinations, 35
    memory, 34–35
    thinking/alertness fluctuations, 35
    visuospatial function, 33–34
  contributing factors, 6–7
  diagnosis, 43
  DLB distinctions from, 13
  dysautonomia in, 37–38
  excessive sleep component, 190–191
  hallmarks of, 5
  name derivation, 13
  nucleus basalis degeneration in, *130,*
    131–132
  parkinsonism of, 36–37
    hospitalization/background for nurses,
      232–234
  pharmacologic treatment guidelines,
    55–57
  psychiatric symptoms in, 39–40
  sleep disorders in, 38–39
  treatment guidelines, 55–57
periodic limb movements of sleep (PLMS),
  188–189
peripheral neuropathy, 107
Petersen, Ronald, 5
pindolol (Visken), 151
Plendil (felodipine), 151
pramipexole (Mirapex), 10, 19, 55, 68, 78
  elimination of, 62
    extended-release, 84
    regular-release, 83–84

hallucinations from, 78, 112
levodopa efficacy comparison, 56–57
pathological behaviors caused by,
117–118, 120
pathologic gambling from, 117–118
in restless legs syndrome, 85, 179
sleepiness induced by, 190
Prinivil (lisinopril), 151
ProAmatine (midodrine), 156–158
Procardia (nifedipine), 151
prochlorperazine (Compazine), 58, 74
prolonged QT syndrome, 206
Prolopa (benserazide and levodopa), 78–79
propranolol (Inderal), 151
Proscan (finasteride), 167
prostate gland
bladder problems and, 161, 163, 165–167
enlargement of
pharmacologic treatment, 152, 167
surgical treatment, 165–166
protriptyline (Vivactil), 153
Provigil (modafinil), 191
Prozac class of medications (SSRIs), 105,
112, 137–138, 178, 201–202
psychiatric symptoms in DLB and PDD. *see*
individual psychiatric symptoms
"pull test" assessment, of balance, 52
pyridostigmine (Mestinon), 158

Q
quetiapine (Seroquel)
for anxiety, 103, 104
dosage strategy, 137
duration of action, 190
for hallucinations, delusions, 113–115,
182, 189
mortality considerations, 104–105, 137
parkinsonism not caused by, 59, 113
sedating properties, 182–183
quinapril (Accupril), 151

R
raloxifene (Evista), 209
ramipril (Altace), 151
rasagiline (MAO-B inhibitor), 20, 55, 56, 68
hallucinations from, 85
interaction with selegiline, 205–206
Razadyne (galantamine), 131, 133–134
Reclast (zoledronic acid), 209
Reglan (metoclopramide), 58, 74
Remeron (mirtazapine), 153
REM sleep behavior disorder
described, 12, 38

differential diagnosis of, 195
as drug side effect, 194
influence on sleep quality, 194–195
information for nurses, 232
melatonin for, 196
in multiple system atrophy, 193–194
risk factors, 195
repetitive movements, impairment of, 50
Requip (ropinirole). *see* ropinirole (Requip)
resting tremor, 10, 36, 52
restless legs syndrome (RLS), 85
drug treatment
carbidopa/levodopa, 179
Mirapex, 117, 179
Neupro, 117, 179
pramipexole/ropinirole, 85, 120, 179
rotigotine, 179
inner restlessness similarity, 183
insomnia caused by, 179
PLMS similarity, 188
rigidity (stiffness), 9–10, 36, 51, 106, 233
risedronate (Actonel, Atelvia), 209
risperidone (Risperdal), 59, 102
Ritalin (methylphenidate), 191
rivastigmine (Exelon)
capsules, 132–133
oral solution, 133
patch, 113, 131, 132
RLS. see restless legs syndrome
Robert Wood Johnson Medical Center, 16
ropinirole (Requip), 10, 55, 68, 78
clinical trials, 19–20
elimination of, for those already taking
medications, 84
levodopa efficacy comparison, 56–57
pathological behaviors caused by,
117–118, 120
pathologic gambling from, 118
possible side effects, 78, 112
in restless legs syndrome, 85
rotigotine potency comparison, 85
sleepiness induced by, 190
rotigotine (Neupro), 10. *see also* Neupro
patch
levodopa efficacy comparison, 56
pathological behaviors caused by, 117–118
possible side effects, 78, 112, 190
in restless legs syndrome, 117, 179
ropinirole potency comparison, 85
sleepiness induced by, 190
slow elimination considerations, 62, 84–85
Rytary (IPX066), investigational carbidopa/
levodopa, 65

S

Sanctura (trospium), 134
selective serotonin reuptake inhibitors
 (SSRIs). *see also* Prozac class of
 medications
 for aggressive behavior, 137–138
 for depression, 112, 178, 200–202
 ECG changes from excess dosage, 206
 insomnia side effect from, 178
 for troublesome thoughts, 105
selegiline (deprenyl) (MAO-B inhibitor), 19,
 55, 56, 68
 hallucinations from, 85
 interaction with rasagiline, 205–206
Seroquel (quetiapine). *see* quetiapine
sexual ideation behavior, from dopamine
 agonists, 119
Short Test of Mental Status, 4
shuffling gait. *see* gait problems
Sinemet (carbidopa/levodopa), 55, 58, 64,
 107
Sinequan (doxepin), 127t, 153, 182, 190, 203
sleep disorders. *see also* daytime drowsiness;
 insomnia; REM sleep behavior
 disorder; restless legs syndrome
 aids for sleep
 anti-hallucination drugs, 182–183
 over-the-counter aids, 181
 quetiapine (Seroquel), 182–183
 sedating antidepressants, 182
 short-acting prescription drugs, 182, 185
 sleep hygiene, 180, 185
 awakening during the night
 from dopamine deficiency, 183–184
 nighttime cramps, 186
 nighttime urination, 184–185
 simple awakening, 185–186
 cognition influenced by, 129
 disturbed sleep architecture, 39
 excessive sleep, 190–191
 insufficient time spent in bed, 186
 periodic limb movements of sleep,
 188–189
 poor quality sleep, 186–187
 sleep apnea, 38, 78, 187–188
smoking compulsivity, from dopamine
 agonists, 118
Sonata (zaleplon), 185
spending behaviors, from dopamine
 agonists, 57, 83, 118, 119
spironolactone (Aldactone), 152
SSRIs. *see* selective serotonin reuptake
 inhibitors

Stalevo (carbidopa/levodopa, entacapone),
 55, 56, 68, 87
stiffness (rigidity), 9–10, 36, 51, 106, 233
stooped posture, 37, 52
stroke, 7, 41, 212, 228
substantia nigra
 degeneration in Lewy body disorders, 28,
 36–37, 49
 location, 27, 28, 28
 role in Parkinson's, DLB, PDD, 28

T

tacrine (Cognex), 131
tamsulosin (Flomax), 167
telmisartan (Micardis), 151
Tenormin (atenolol), 151
terazosin (Hytrin), 152, 167
teriparatide (Forteo), 209
thinking fluctuations, in DLB and PDD. *see*
 cognition; delusions; dementia
Tiazac (diltiazem), 151
Tigan (trimethobenzamide), 58, 74
timolol (Blocadren), 151
Tofranil (imipramine), 153
tolcapone (COMT inhibitor), 87
Toprol (metoprolol), 151
torsemide (Demadex), 152
treatment options for those already on
 medications, 81–88
 amantadine, 86
 anticholinergics, elimination of
 benztropine (Cogentin), 82–83
 trihexyphenidyl (Artane), 82–83
 combination side effects, 81–82
 COMT inhibitors, 86–87
 dopamine agonists, elimination of
 pramipexole (Mirapex), extended
 release, 84
 pramipexole (Mirapex), regular release,
 83–84
 ropinirole (Requip), regular-release, 84
 ropinirole (Requip XL), extended
 release, 84
 rotigotine patch (Neupro), 84–85
tremors
 essential tremor, 36, 53, 151
 Lewy ("at rest") tremor, 10, 36, 52
triamterene (with HCTZ, Dyazide), 152
tricyclic antidepressants, 127t, 153, 169–170,
 200
trihexyphenidyl (Artane), 57, 68,
 82–83
trimethobenzamide (Tigan), 58, 74

trospium (Sanctura), 134
Tylenol PM (acetaminophen and
    diphenhydramine), 181

U
urinary hesitancy, 161, 163, 165–166
urinary tract infections (UTIs), 113, 115,
    128, 163–167, 236
  bladder problems and, 163
  cognitive decompensations from, 128
  diagnosis, 166–167
  hallucinations from, 112–113, 115
  neurologic decline from, 167
  treatment, 166–167
urinary urge incontinence, 164–165
Uroxatral (alfuzosin), 167
U.S. Food and Drug Administration (FDA)
  Advisory Panel rasagiline report, 20
  memantine approval for Alzheimer's, 134
  neuroleptic drug warning, 114–115
  pending Rytary approval, 65

V
Valium (diazepam), 102, 127*t*, 189*t*, 190
Valium class of medications. *see also*
    benzodiazepines
  for aggression, acting out, 137
  for anxiety, 102
  quetiapine comparison, 137

for REM sleep behavior, 196
  side effects of, 112, 137
valsartan (Diovan), 151
Vasotec (enalapril), 151
verapamil (Calan, Isoptin, Verelan), 151
Verelan (verapamil), 151
Visken (pindolol), 151
visuospatial function, in DLB and PDD,
    33–34
Vivactil (protriptyline), 153
volitional movements, 26

W
walking difficulties, x–xi, 10, 36, 51, 207
water pills (diuretics), 147, 152, 164, 184, 234
writing movements, 26

X
Xanax (alprazolam), 102, 127*t*, 137, 189*t*, 235

Z
zaleplon (Sonata), 185
Zestril (lisinopril), 151
ziprasidone (Geodon), 102
Zofran (ondansetron), 58, 74
zoledronic acid (Reclast, Zometa), 209
zolpidem (Ambien), 185
Zometa (zoledronic acid), 209
Zyprexa (olanzapine), 102

Printed in the USA/Agawam, MA
March 23, 2017

649754.013